Vagus Nerve

Learn how to activate your natural healing power trough exercise for reducing inflammations, depression, trauma, anxiety.

© **Copyright 2019 by Susanne Moriarty**
All rights reserved.

This document is geared towards providing exact and reliable information with regards to the topic and issue covered. The publication is sold with the idea that the publisher is not required to render accounting, officially permitted, or otherwise, qualified services. If advice is necessary, legal or professional, a practiced individual in the profession should be ordered.

- From a Declaration of Principles which was accepted and approved equally by a Committee of the American Bar Association and a Committee of Publishers and Associations.

In no way is it legal to reproduce, duplicate, or transmit any part of this document in either electronic means or in printed format. Recording of this publication is strictly prohibited and any storage of this document is not allowed unless with written permission from the publisher. All rights reserved.

The information provided herein is stated to be truthful and consistent, in that any liability, in terms of inattention or otherwise, by any usage or abuse of any policies, processes, or directions contained within is the solitary and utter responsibility of the recipient reader. Under no circumstances will any legal responsibility or blame be held against the publisher for any reparation, damages, or monetary loss due to the information herein, either directly or indirectly.

Respective authors own all copyrights not held by the publisher.

The information herein is offered for informational purposes solely, and is universal as so. The presentation of the information is without contract or any type of guarantee assurance.

The trademarks that are used are without any consent, and the publication of the trademark is without permission or backing by the trademark owner. All trademarks and brands within this book are for clarifying purposes only and are the owned by the owners themselves, not affiliated with this document

Table of Contents

Chapter One: Vagus Nerve anatomy disclosure...... 1

What is the vagus nerve? 1

Vagus nerve life structures and capacity 2

Vagus nerve testing 3

Vagus nerve issues 4

    Nerve harm 4

Gastroparesis 5

Vasovagal syncope 6

Vagus nerve incitement 6

What is the vagus nerve? 7

What does the vagus nerve influence? 8

Vagus Nerve Outburst 11

Epilepsy 11

Psychological maladjustment 13

Chapter Two: Nine realities about this amazing nerve group. 16

1. THE VAGUS NERVE PREVENTS INFLAMMATION. 16

2. IT HELPS YOU MAKE MEMORIES 17

3. IT HELPS YOU BREATHE 17

4. IT'S INTIMATELY INVOLVED WITH YOUR HEART. 18

5. IT INITIATES YOUR BODY'S RELAXATION RESPONSE. 18

6. IT TRANSLATES BETWEEN YOUR GUT AND YOUR BRAIN 19

7. OVERSTIMULATION OF THE VAGUS NERVE IS THE MOST COMMON CAUSE OF FAINTING. 19

8. ELECTRICAL STIMULATION OF THE VAGUS NERVE REDUCES INFLAMMATION AND MAY INHIBIT IT ALTOGETHER. 20

9. VAGUS NERVE STIMULATION HAS CREATED A NEW FIELD OF MEDICINE. 21

Comprehension 23

Essential Anatomy of the Vagus Nerve 24

Elements of the Vagus Nerve.. 27

Vagus Nerve as Modulator of Intestinal Immune Homeostasis 35

Vagus Nerve Stimulation 38

Gadget and Method..38

The Neural Mechanism of VNS 40

Vagus-Related Treatment of Depression 45

    Essential Pathophysiology of Depression.................... 45

VNS in Depression 46

Impact of Nutrition Depressive Symptoms 48

Vagus-Related Treatment of PTSD 52

    Pathophysiology of PTSD... 52

VNS in PTSD.. 56

Positive Influence of Nutritive Components on PTSD ... 58

Positive Influence of Meditation and Yoga on PTSD 59

Vagus-Related Treatment of PTSD 62

    Pathophysiology of PTSD... 62

VNS in PTSD.. 66

Positive Influence of Nutritive Components on PTSD ... 68

Positive Influence of Meditation and Yoga on PTSD 69

Chapter Three: How is it composed, and how does it work? 73

Life structures of the Vagus Nerve 73

The capacity of the Vagus Nerve 74

The Vasovagal Reflex 75

The Vagus Nerve and the Heart 76

The Vagus Nerve in Medical Therapy 76

Why the Vagus Nerve is so Important 78

How might you bolster your vagus nerve? 81

Chapter Four: The functions of the vagus nerve ... 83

Anatomical Course 83

In the Head 83

In the Neck 84

In the Thorax 85

In the Abdomen 86

Tactile Functions 86

Uncommon Sensory Functions 87

The benefits of Vagus Nerve By Kelly 90

Vagus Nerve as a Link between the Central and ENS .. 100

The mind-gut pivot 103

Vagus nerve incitement as a restorative treatment 105

Harm to the vagus nerve 106

The vagus nerve and blacking out 107

Resting and processing 110

When is VNS used to treat epilepsy? 113

IT'S CLICHE, BUT TAKE DEEP BREATHS 116

KEEP YOUR GUT HAPPY 118

Discover YOUR SAFETY CUES 120

Utilize SOOTHING VOICES 121
TRAIN YOUR OWN SAFETY CUES 122
Deal with YOUR MYELIN 123
YOU CAN TONE YOUR BABY'S VAGUS NERVE 124
How does the vagus nerve influence wellbeing? 128
What causes your vagus nerve to fail to meet expectations. 129
Barriers to Vagus Nerve while functioning 138

Chapter Five: Relations between vagus nerves and parasympathetic system 140

Step by step instructions to Hack Your Nervous System 140
The longest cranial nerve vagus nerve is the longest of our 12 cranial nerves. 144
Structure of the Parasympathetic Limb of the Autonomic Nervous System 146
Parasympathetic/Sympathetic Interactions 148
Muscarinic Receptors 150
Nicotinic Receptors 152
Sorts of Vagus Nerve Fibers 153
Focal Influences on Parasympathetic Innervation 155
Pulse Control 156
Pulse and Outcomes 156
Assessment of Parasympathetic Activation 157
Change of Parasympathetic Control in HF 159

Chapter Six: How to treat symptoms naturally ... 162

Dangers 165
Medical procedure dangers 165
How you plan 167

Nourishment and drugs 167

What you can anticipate 167

During the technique 168

Vagus Nerve Stimulation (VNS) Dramatically Reduces Arthritic Inflammation 176

How improving your vagal tone can prevent physical inflammation 179

Chapter Seven: Vagus nerve stimulation routine you can add to your daily habit 188

Ice 197

Chapter Eight: How to strengthen Vagus Nerve . 198

Yoga Self-Care 198

Slow, Deep, Breathing 200

Exercise 201

Metta Meditation 201

Brief Recitation 202

Nineteen efficient ways to Improve Vagal Tone 205

Chapter One: Vagus Nerve anatomy disclosure

What is the vagus nerve?

There are 12 cranial nerves in the body. They come two by two and help to interface the mind with different regions of the body, for example, the head, neck, and middle. Some send tactile data, including insights concerning smells, sights, tastes, and sounds, to the cerebrum. These nerves are known as having tangible capacities. Other cranial nerves control the development of different muscles and the capacity of specific organs. These are known as engine capacities. While some cranial nerves have either tangible or engine capacities, others have both. The vagus nerve is such a nerve. The cranial nerves are grouped utilizing Roman numerals dependent on their area. The vagus nerve is likewise called cranial nerve X. The substantial ways of deciphering vagus nerve are as follows:

Vagus nerve life structures and capacity

"Vagus" signifies meandering in Latin. This is a fitting name, as the vagus nerve is the longest cranial nerve. It runs right from the cerebrum stem to part of the colon.

The tangible elements of the vagus nerve are partitioned into two segments:

- Substantial segments. These are sensations felt on the skin or in the muscles.
- Instinctive segments. These are sensations felt in the organs of the body.

Tangible elements of the vagus nerve include:

Giving substantial sensation data to the skin behind the ear, the outer piece of the ear trench, and certain pieces of the throat providing instinctive sensation data for the larynx, throat, lungs, trachea, heart, and the vast majority of the stomach related tract assuming a little job in the impression of taste close to the base of the tongue

Engine elements of the vagus nerve include:

- invigorating muscles in the pharynx, larynx, and the delicate sense of taste, which is the plump zone close the back of the top of the mouth
- animating muscles in the heart, where it brings down resting pulse
- animating automatic constrictions in the stomach related tract, including the throat, stomach, and the vast majority of the digestive organs, which enable nourishment to travel through the tract

Vagus nerve testing

To test the vagus nerve, a specialist may check the muffle reflex. During this piece of the assessment, the specialist may utilize a delicate cotton swab to tickle the back of the throat on the two sides. This should make the individual stifler. In the event that the individual doesn't choke, this might be because of an issue with the vagus nerve.

Vagus nerve issues

Nerve harm

Harm to the vagus nerve can have a scope of side effects in light of the fact that the nerve is so long and influences numerous regions.

Potential side effects of harm to the vagus nerve include:

- trouble talking or loss of voice
- a voice that is rough or wheezy
- inconvenience drinking fluids
- loss of the muffle reflex
- torment in the ear
- bizarre pulse
- anomalous circulatory strain
- diminished creation of stomach corrosive
- queasiness or regurgitating
- stomach swelling or torment

The side effects somebody may have to rely upon what some portion of the nerve is harmed.

Gastroparesis

Specialists accept that harm to the vagus nerve may likewise cause a condition called gastroparesis. This condition influences the automatic withdrawals of the stomach related framework, which keeps the stomach from appropriately exhausting.

Indications of gastroparesis include:

- queasiness or heaving, particularly retching undigested nourishment hours subsequent to eating
- loss of craving or feeling full not long after beginning a feast
- heartburn
- stomach torment or swelling
- unexplained weight reduction
- variances in glucose

A few people create gastroparesis in the wake of experiencing a vagotomy method, which evacuates all or part of the vagus nerve.

Vasovagal syncope

Now and then the vagus nerve goes overboard to certain pressure triggers, for example,

- introduction to outrageous warmth
- the dread of substantial damage
- seeing blood or having blood drawn
- stressing, including attempting to having a solid discharge
- representing quite a while

Keep in mind; the vagus nerve animates certain muscles in the heart that help to slow pulse. At the point when it goes overboard, it can cause an unexpected drop in pulse and circulatory strain, bringing about blacking out. This is known as vasovagal syncope.

Vagus nerve incitement

Vagus nerve incitement includes setting a gadget in the body that utilizations electrical driving forces to reenact the nerve. It's utilized to treat a few instances of epilepsy and sorrow that don't react to different medicines.

The gadget is typically put under the skin of the chest, where a wire interfaces it to one side vagus nerve. When the gadget is initiated, it sends a flag through the vagus nerve to your brainstem, which at that point, transmits data to your cerebrum. A nervous system specialist as a rule program the gadget; however, individuals frequently get a handheld magnet they can use to control the gadget all alone also.

It's the idea that vagus nerve incitement could treat a scope of different conditions later on, including various sclerosisTrusted Source, Alzheimer's disease, Trusted Source, and bunch headaches trusted Sources.

What is the vagus nerve?

The vagus nerve is one of the cranial nerves that interface the mind to the body.

The vagus nerve has two lots of tactile nerve cell bodies, and it interfaces the brainstem to the body. It enables the cerebrum to screen and get data around a few of the body's various capacities.

There are different sensory system capacities gave by the vagus nerve and its related parts. The vagus nerve capacities add to the autonomic sensory system, which comprises of the parasympathetic and thoughtful parts. The nerve is answerable for certain tangible exercises and engine data for development inside the body.

Basically, it is a piece of a circuit that connections the neck, heart, lungs, and stomach area to the cerebrum.

What does the vagus nerve influence?

The vagus nerve has various capacities. The four key elements of the vagus nerve are:

- Tactile: From the throat, heart, lungs, and belly.
- Exceptional tactile: Provides taste sensation behind the tongue.
- Engine: Provides development capacities for the muscles in the neck answerable for gulping and discourse.

- Parasympathetic: Responsible for the stomach related tract, breath, and pulse working.

Its capacities can be separated significantly further into seven classifications. One of these is adjusting the sensory system.

The sensory system can be separated into two regions: thoughtful and parasympathetic. The thoughtful side expands readiness, vitality, circulatory strain, pulse, and breathing rate.

The parasympathetic side, which the vagus nerve is intensely associated with, diminishes readiness, circulatory strain, and pulse, and assists with smoothness, unwinding, and assimilation. Therefore, the vagus nerve likewise assists with crap, pee, and sexual excitement.

Different vagus nerve impacts include:

Correspondence between the cerebrum and the gut: The vagus nerve conveys data from the gut to the mind.

- Unwinding with profound breathing: The vagus nerve speaks with the stomach. With full breaths, an individual feels increasingly loose.
- Diminishing irritation: The vagus nerve sends a mitigating sign to different pieces of the body.
- Bringing down the pulse and circulatory strain: If the vagus nerve is overactive, it can prompt the heart being not able to siphon enough blood around the body. At times, unnecessary vagus nerve action can cause loss of awareness and organ harm.
- Dread administration: The vagus nerve sends data from the gut to the cerebrum, which is connected to managing pressure, nervousness, and dread - thus the maxim, "hunch." These sign assistance an individual to recuperate from upsetting and frightening circumstances.

Vagus Nerve Outburst

The incitement of the vagus nerve is a medicinal strategy that is utilized to attempt to treat an assortment of conditions. It very well may be done either physically or through electrical heartbeats.

The adequacy of vagus nerve incitement has been tried through clinical preliminaries. Subsequently, the United States Food and Drug Administration (FDA)Trusted Source had affirmed its utilization to treat two unique conditions.

Epilepsy

In 1997, the FDA permitted the utilization of vagus nerve incitement for hard-headed epilepsy.

This includes a little electrical gadget, like a pacemaker, being put in an individual's chest. A slight wire known as a lead runs from the gadget to the vagus nerve.

The gadget is set in the body by the medical procedure under a general sedative. It, at that point, sends electrical driving forces at standard interims, for the duration of the day, to the mind by means of the vagus nerve to diminish the seriousness, or even stop, seizures.

Vagus nerve incitement for epilepsy may have some symptoms, including sore throat and trouble gulping.

Symptoms of vagus nerve incitement for epilepsy include:

- raspiness or changes in voice
- sore throat
- brevity of breath
- hacking
- slow pulse
- trouble gulping
- stomach uneasiness or queasiness

Individuals utilizing this type of treatment ought to consistently tell their primary care physician in the event that they are having any issues as there might be approaches to lessen or stop these.

Psychological maladjustment

In 2005, the FDA endorsed the utilization of vagus nerve incitement as a treatment for melancholy. It has likewise been found to help trusted Source with the accompanying conditions:

- quick cycling bipolar issue
- tension issue
- Alzheimer's ailment

With the vagus nerve having pathways to pretty much every organ in the body, analysts are hoping to check whether incitement can support different conditions.

Studies propose that incitement of the vagus nerve may lessen the side effects of rheumatoid joint inflammation.

These conditions include:

- rheumatoid joint inflammation irritation
- cardiovascular breakdown
- irritation from diabetes mellitus
- recalcitrant hiccups

- strange heart mood
- irritation from Crohn's illness

On account of rheumatoid joint inflammation, which influences 1.3 million grown-ups in the U.S., an examination in 2016 demonstrated that vagus nerve incitement could help decrease side effects. People who had neglected to react to other treatment detailed huge upgrades, while no genuine unfavorable symptoms were noted.

This was viewed as a genuine leap forward in how vagus nerve incitement may regard rheumatoid joint pain as well as other fiery sicknesses, for example, Crohn's, Parkinson's, and Alzheimer's.

The vagus nerve is so named in light of the fact that it "meanders" like a drifter, conveying tactile filaments from your brainstem to your instinctive organs. The vagus nerve, the longest of the cranial nerves, controls your inward operational hub—the parasympathetic sensory system. Also, it directs a tremendous scope of vital capacities, conveying engine, and tangible motivations to each organ in your body. New research has uncovered that it might likewise be the missing connect to treating constant irritation, and the start of an energizing new field of treatment for genuine, serious ailments.

Chapter Two: Nine realities about this amazing nerve group.

1. THE VAGUS NERVE PREVENTS INFLAMMATION.

A specific measure of irritation after damage or ailment is ordinary. Yet, an excess is connected to numerous illnesses and conditions, from sepsis to the immune system condition rheumatoid joint inflammation. The vagus nerve works an immense system of strands positioned like covert agents around the entirety of your organs. At the point when it gets a sign for nascent aggravation—the nearness of cytokines or a substance called tumor corruption factor (TNF)— it alarms the cerebrum and draws out calming synapses that manage the body's resistant reaction.

2. IT HELPS YOU MAKE MEMORIES.

A University of Virginia study in rodents demonstrated that animating their vagus nerves reinforced their memory. The activity discharged the synapse norepinephrine into the amygdala, which solidified recollections. Related investigations were done in people, proposing promising medications for conditions like Alzheimer's malady.

3. IT HELPS YOU BREATHE.

The synapse acetylcholine, evoked by the vagus nerve, advises your lungs to relax. It's one reason that Botox—frequently utilized cosmetically—can be conceivably perilous, in light of the fact that it intrudes on your acetylcholine creation. You can, in any case, additionally invigorate your vagus nerve by doing stomach breathing or holding your breath for four to eight tallies.

4. IT'S INTIMATELY INVOLVED WITH YOUR HEART.

The vagus nerve is answerable for controlling the pulse by means of electrical driving forces to specific muscle tissue—the heart's characteristic pacemaker—in the correct chamber, where acetylcholine discharge eases back the beat. By estimating the time between your individual heart thumps, and afterward plotting this on an outline over the long run, specialists can decide your pulse changeability or HRV. This information can offer signs about the versatility of your heart and vagus nerve.

5. IT INITIATES YOUR BODY'S RELAXATION RESPONSE.

When your ever-careful thoughtful sensory system fires up the battle or flight reactions—pouring the pressure hormone cortisol and adrenaline into your body—the vagus nerve advises your body to relax by discharging acetylcholine. The vagus nerve's ringlets stretch out to numerous organs, acting like fiber-optic links that send guidelines to discharge catalysts and proteins like prolactin, vasopressin, and oxytocin, which quiet you down. Individuals with a more grounded vagus reaction might be bound to recuperate all the more rapidly after pressure, damage, or sickness.

6. IT TRANSLATES BETWEEN YOUR GUT AND YOUR BRAIN.

Your gut utilizes the vagus nerve like a walkie-talkie to tell your cerebrum how you're feeling by means of electric motivations called "activity possibilities." Your premonitions are genuine.

7. OVERSTIMULATION OF THE VAGUS NERVE IS THE MOST COMMON CAUSE OF FAINTING.

On the off chance that you tremble or get nauseous at seeing blood or while getting an influenza shot, you're not frail. You're encountering, "vagal syncope." Your body, reacting to pressure, overstimulates the vagus nerve, causing your circulatory strain and pulse to drop. During outrageous syncope, the bloodstream is limited to your cerebrum, and you lose cognizance. However, more often than not, you simply need to sit or rests for the side effects of dying down.

8. ELECTRICAL STIMULATION OF THE VAGUS NERVE REDUCES INFLAMMATION AND MAY INHIBIT IT ALTOGETHER.

Neurosurgeon Kevin Tracey was the first to show that animating the vagus nerve can essentially decrease irritation. Results on rodents were so fruitful. He imitated the investigation in people with staggering outcomes. The formation of inserts to invigorate the vagus nerve by means of electronic inserts demonstrated a radical decrease, and even abatement, in rheumatoid joint pain—which has no known fix and is regularly treated with the poisonous medications—hemorrhagic stun, and other similarly genuine fiery disorders.

9. VAGUS NERVE STIMULATION HAS CREATED A NEW FIELD OF MEDICINE.

Prodded on by the accomplishment of vagal nerve incitement to treat aggravation and epilepsy, a thriving field of restorative examination, known as bioelectronics, might be the fate of medication. Utilizing inserts that convey electric motivations to different body parts, researchers and specialists would like to treat sickness with fewer prescriptions and fewer reactions.

Why it is the most important nerve in your body

The vagus nerve speaks to the fundamental segment of the parasympathetic sensory system, which manages a huge range of substantial vital capacities, including control of temperament, insusceptible reaction, processing, and pulse. It builds up one of the associations between the mind and the gastrointestinal tract and sends data about the condition of the internal organs to the cerebrum through afferent filaments. In this survey research, we talk about different elements of the vagus nerve which make it an alluring objective in treating the mental and gastrointestinal issues. There is starter proof that vagus nerve incitement is a promising extra treatment for treatment-recalcitrant sadness, posttraumatic stress issues, and fiery inside ailment. Medications that focus on the vagus nerve increment the vagal tone and hinder cytokine creation. Both are a significant system of flexibility. The incitement of vagal afferent strands in the gut impacts monoaminergic cerebrum frameworks in the mind stem that assume essential jobs in major mental conditions, for example, disposition and nervousness issue. Inline, there is fundamental proof for gut microbes to have advantageous impact on mind-set and uneasiness, halfway by influencing the action of the vagus nerve. Since the vagal tone is related to the ability to manage pressure reactions and can be affected by breathing, its expansion through reflection and yoga likely adds to flexibility and the alleviation of disposition and uneasiness side effects.

Comprehension

The bidirectional correspondence between the cerebrum and the gastrointestinal tract, the alleged "mind-gut pivot," depends on a perplexing framework, including the vagus nerve, yet in addition thoughtful (e.g., by means of the prevertebral ganglia), endocrine, insusceptible, and humoral connections just as the impact of gut microbiota so as to direct gastrointestinal homeostasis and to interface enthusiastic and subjective territories of the mind with gut capacities . The ENS delivers in excess of 30 synapses and has a larger number of neurons than the spine. Hormones and peptides that the ENS discharges into the blood course cross the blood–cerebrum boundary (e.g., ghrelin) and can act synergistically with the vagus nerve, for instance, to manage nourishment admission and hunger. The mind-gut pivot is getting progressively significant as a helpful objective for gastrointestinal and mental issues, for example, fiery inside ailment (IBD), misery, and posttraumatic stress issues (PTSD). The gut is a significant control focal point of the invulnerable framework, and the vagus nerve has immunomodulatory properties. Thus, this nerve assumes significant jobs in the connection between the gut, the cerebrum, and irritation. There are new treatment choices for tweaking the cerebrum gut hub, for instance, vagus nerve incitement (VNS) and reflection systems. These medications have been demonstrated to be helpful in state of mind and tension issue, yet in addition to different conditions related to expanded aggravation. Specifically, gut-coordinated hypnotherapy was demonstrated to be successful in both, touchy entrail disorder and IBD. At long last, the vagus nerve additionally speaks to a significant connection among nourishment and mental, neurological and incendiary infections.

Essential Anatomy of the Vagus Nerve

The vagus nerve conveys a broad scope of signs from stomach related framework and organs to the mind and the other way around. It is the tenth cranial nerve, reaching out from its starting point in the brainstem through the neck and the thorax down to the stomach area. In view of its long way through the human body, it has likewise been depicted as the "vagabond nerve."

The vagus nerve exits from the medulla oblongata, ready between the olive and the substandard cerebellar peduncle, leaving the skull through the center compartment of the jugular foramen. In the neck, the vagus nerve gives expected innervation to the vast majority of the muscles of the pharynx and larynx, which are liable for gulping and vocalization. In the thorax, it gives the primary parasympathetic stockpile to the heart and invigorates a decrease in the pulse. In the digestive organs, the vagus nerve directs the constriction of smooth muscles and glandular discharge. Preganglionic neurons of vagal efferent filaments rise up out of the dorsal engine core of the vagus nerve situated in the medulla and innervate the solid and mucosal layers of the gut both in the lamina propria. The celiac branch supplies the digestive system from proximal duodenum to the distal piece of the slipping colon. The stomach vagal afferents, incorporate mucosal mechanoreceptors, chemoreceptors, and strain receptors in the throat, stomach, and proximal small digestive tract, and tangible endings in the liver and pancreas. The tangible afferent cell bodies are situated in nodose ganglia and send data to the core tractus solitarii (NTS). The NTS extends, the vagal tactile data to a few locales of the CNS, for example, the locus coeruleus (LC), the rostral ventrolateral medulla, the amygdala, and the thalamus.

The vagus nerve is answerable for the guideline of inside organ capacities, for example, processing, pulse, and respiratory rate, just as vasomotor movement, and certain reflex activities, for example, hacking, sniffling, gulping, and retching. Its actuation prompts the arrival of acetylcholine (ACh) at the synaptic intersection with discharging cells, characteristic apprehensive strands, and smooth muscles. ACh ties to nicotinic and muscarinic receptors and animates muscle constrictions in the parasympathetic sensory system.

Creature ponders shown a striking recovery limit of the vagus nerve. For instance, subdiaphragmatic vagotomy prompted transient withdrawal and rebuilding of focal vagal afferents just as synaptic versatility in the NTS. Further, the recovery of vagal afferents in rodents can be arrived at 18 weeks after subdiaphragmatic vagotomy, despite the fact that the efferent reinnervation of the gastrointestinal tract isn't reestablished much following 45 weeks.

Elements of the Vagus Nerve

The Role of Vagus in the Functions of the Autonomic Nervous System

Close by the thoughtful sensory system and the enteric sensory system (ENS), the parasympathetic sensory system speaks to one of the three parts of the autonomic sensory system.

The meaning of thoughtful and parasympathetic sensory systems is fundamentally anatomical. The vagus nerve is the fundamental benefactor of the parasympathetic sensory system. The other three parasympathetic cranial nerves are the nervus oculomotorius, the nervus facialis, and the nervus glossopharyngeus.

The most significant capacity of the vagus nerve is afferent, bringing data of the inward organs, for example, gut, liver, heart, and lungs to the cerebrum. This recommends the inward organs are significant wellsprings of tangible data to the mind. The gut as the biggest surface toward the external world and might, in this manner, be an especially significant tactile organ.

Generally, the vagus has been considered as an efferent nerve and as a rival of the thoughtful sensory system. Most organs get parasympathetic efferents through the vagus nerve and thoughtful efferents through the splanchnic nerves. Together with the thoughtful sensory systems, the parasympathetic sensory system is liable for the guideline of vegetative capacities by acting contrary to one another. The parasympathetic innervation causes dilatation of veins and bronchioles and incitement of salivary organs. Despite what might be expected, the thoughtful innervation prompts a narrowing of veins, a dilatation of bronchioles, an expansion in pulse, and a choking of intestinal and urinary sphincters. In the gastrointestinal tract, the actuation of the parasympathetic sensory system expands gut motility and glandular discharge. Rather than it, the thoughtful movement prompts a decrease of intestinal action and a decrease of bloodstream to the gut, permitting a higher bloodstream to the heart and the muscles, when the individual faces existential pressure.

The ENS emerges from neural peak cells of the fundamentally vagal root and comprises of a nerve plexus inserted in the intestinal divider, reaching out over the entire gastrointestinal tract from the throat to the butt. It is evaluated that the human ENS contains around 100–500 million neurons. This is the biggest aggregation of nerve cells in the human body. Since the ENS is like the cerebrum in regards to structure, capacity, and substance coding, it has been depicted as "the subsequent mind" or "the cerebrum inside the gut." It comprises two ganglionated plexuses—the submucosal plexus, which directs gastrointestinal bloodstream and controls the epithelial cell capacities and emission and the myenteric plexus, which for the most part manages the unwinding and withdrawal of the intestinal divider. The ENS fills in as an intestinal obstruction and controls the major enteric procedures, for example, resistant reaction, recognizing supplements, motility, microvascular flow, and epithelial emission of liquids, particles, and bioactive peptides. There unmistakably is "correspondence" between the vagal nerve and the ENS, and the principle transmitter is cholinergic enactment through nicotinic receptors. The connection of ENS and the vagal nerve as a piece of the CNS prompts a bidirectional progression of data. Then again, the ENS in the little and enormous inside additionally can work very free of vagal control as it contains full reflex circuits, including tangible neurons and engine neurons. They direct muscle movement and motility, liquid motions, mucosal bloodstream, and furthermore mucosal boundary work.

Cholecystokinin directs gastrointestinal capacities, including restraint of gastric purging and nourishment consumption through the enactment of CCK-1 receptors on vagal afferent strands innervating the gut. Furthermore, CCK is significant for the emission of pancreatic liquid and creating gastric corrosive, getting the gallbladder, diminishing gastric purging, and encouraging absorption (. Immersed fat, long-chain unsaturated fats, amino acids, and little peptides that outcome from protein processing invigorates the arrival of CCK from the small digestive system. There are different organically dynamic types of CCK, ordered by the number of amino acids they contain, i.e., CCK-5, CCK-8, CCK-22, and CCK-33. In neurons, CCK-8 is consistently the prevailing structure, though the endocrine gut cells contain a blend of little and bigger CCK peptides of which CCK-33 or CCK-22 regularly prevail. In rodents, both long-and short-chain unsaturated fats from nourishment actuate jejunal vagal afferent nerve filaments, however, do as such by unmistakable components. Short-chain unsaturated fats, for example, butyric corrosive directly affect vagal afferent terminals while the long-chain unsaturated fats enact vagal afferents by means of a CCK-subordinate instrument. The exogenous organization of CCK seems to repress endogenous CCK discharge. CCK is likewise present in enteric vagal afferent neurons, in the cerebral cortex, in the thalamus, nerve center, basal ganglia, and dorsal hindbrain, and capacities as a synapse. It straightforwardly initiates vagal afferent terminals in the NTS by expanding calcium discharge. Further, there is proof that CCK can enact neurons in the hindbrain and myenteric intestinal plexus (a plexus which gives engine innervation to the two layers of the solid layer of the gut), in rodents and that vagotomy or capsaicin treatment brings about a lessening of CCK-actuated Fo's articulation (a sort of a proto-oncogene) in mind (There is likewise considerable proof that raised degrees of CCK to incite sentiments of nervousness . Along these lines, CCK is utilized as a test operator to show tension issues in people and creatures.

Ghrelin is another hormone discharged into dissemination from the stomach and assumes a key job in animating nourishment consumption by repressing vagal afferent terminating. Circling ghrelin levels are expanded by fasting and fall after dinner. Focal or fringe organization of acylated ghrelin to rodents intensely animates nourishment admission and development hormone discharge, and incessant organization causes weight increase. The activity of ghrelin's on nourishing is abrogated or constricted in rodents that have experienced vagotomy or treatment with capsaicin, a particular afferent neurotoxin. In people, intravenous imbuement or subcutaneous infusion increments the two sentiments of craving and nourishment consumption, since ghrelin stifles insulin discharge. In this manner, it isn't astounding that emission is upset in stoutness and insulin obstruction.

Leptin receptors have additionally been distinguished in the vagus nerve. Concentrates in rodents obviously show that leptin and CCK collaborate synergistically to instigate momentary restraint of nourishment to allow and long haul decrease of body weight. The epithelial cells that react to both ghrelin and leptin are situated close to the vagal mucosal endings and adjust the action of vagal afferents, acting in the show to control nourishment consumption. Subsequent to fasting and diet-actuated heftiness in mice, leptin loses its potentiating impact on vagal mucosal afferents.

The gastrointestinal tract is the key interface among nourishment and the human body and can detect essential preferences for similarly as the tongue, using comparable G-protein-coupled taste receptors. Distinctive taste characteristics actuate the arrival of various gastric peptides. Unpleasant taste receptors can be considered as potential focuses to lessen hunger by animating the arrival of CCK. Further, the actuation of unpleasant taste receptors invigorates ghrelin emission and, hence, influences the vagus nerve.

Vagus Nerve as Modulator of Intestinal Immune Homeostasis

The gastrointestinal tract is continually gone up against with nourishment antigens, potential pathogens, and advantageous intestinal microbiota that present a hazard factor for intestinal irritation. It is profoundly innervated by vagal strands that associate the CNS with the invulnerable intestinal framework, making vagus a significant part, the neuroendocrine-safe pivot. This pivot is engaged with facilitated neural, social, and endocrine reactions, significant for the principal line barrier against irritation. For instance, in light of pathogens and different harmful boosts, tumor-putrefaction factor-alpha (TNF-α), a cytokine, is delivered by initiated macrophages, dendritic cells, and different cells in the mucosa. Together with prostaglandins and interferons, TNF-α is a significant middle person of the neighborhood and foundational irritation and expands causing the cardinal clinical indications of aggravation, including heat, growing torment, and redness. Counter-administrative instruments, for example, immunologically capable cells and calming cytokines, ordinarily limit the intense provocative reaction and anticipate the spread of fiery arbiters into the circulatory system. Further, there is a "hard-wired" association between the apprehensive and the insusceptible framework that works as a mitigating system. The dorsal vagal complex, containing the tangible cores of the single track, the region postrema, and the dorsal engine core of the vagus, reacts to expanded coursing measures of TNF-α by changing engine action in the vagus nerve.

The calming limits of the vagus nerve are intervened through three unique pathways. The primary pathway is the HPA pivot, which has been depicted previously. The subsequent pathway is the splenic thoughtful mitigating pathway, where the vagus nerve animates the thoughtful splenic nerve. Norepinephrine (NE) (noradrenaline) discharged at the distal finish of the splenic nerve connects to the β2 adrenergic receptor of splenic lymphocytes that discharge ACh. At long last, ACh hinders the arrival of TNF-α by spleen macrophages through α-7-nicotinic ACh receptors. The last pathway, called the mitigating cholinergic pathway (CAIP), is interceded through vagal efferent strands that neurotransmitter onto enteric neurons, which thus discharge ACh at the synaptic intersection with macrophages. ACh ties to α-7-nicotinic ACh receptors of those macrophages to repress the TNF-α. Contrasted with the HPA hub, the CAIP has some interesting properties, for example, a fast of neural conductance, which empowers a quick modulatory contribution to the influenced area of irritation. Consequently, the CAIP assumes an urgent job in the intestinal invulnerable reaction and homeostasis and presents a profoundly intriguing objective for the improvement of novel medications for fiery sicknesses identified with the gut safe framework.

The irritation detecting and aggravation smothering capacities laid out above give the vital parts of the incendiary reflex. The presence of pathogenic life forms enacts natural invulnerable cells that discharge cytokines. These thusly actuate tactile filaments that rise in the vagus nerve to neural connection in the core tractus solitarius. Expanded efferent flag in the vagus nerve smothers fringe cytokine discharge through macrophage nicotinic receptors and the CAIP. Therefore, exploratory enactment of the CAIP by direct electrical incitement of the efferent vagus nerve restrains the amalgamation of TNF-α in the liver, spleen, and heart, and weakens serum convergences of TNF-α.

Vagus Nerve Stimulation

Vagus nerve incitement is a restorative treatment that is routinely utilized in the treatment of epilepsy and other neurological conditions. VNS considers are clinically, yet in addition, experimentally instructive in regards to the job of the vagus nerve in wellbeing and infection.

Gadget and Method

Vagus nerve incitement works by applying electrical motivations to the vagus nerve. The incitement of the vagus nerve can be performed in two unique manners: a direct obtrusive incitement, which is, as of now, the most continuous application and an aberrant transcutaneous non-intrusive incitement. Obtrusive VNS (iVNS) requires the careful implantation of a little heartbeat generator subcutaneously in the left thoracic locale. Terminals are joined to one side cervical vagus nerve and are associated with the heartbeat generator by a lead, which is burrowed under the skin. The generator conveys irregular electrical driving forces through the vagus nerve to the mind. It is hypothesized that these electrical driving forces apply antiepileptic, upper, and calming impacts by changing the edginess of nerve cells. Rather than iVNS, transcutaneous VNS (tVNS) considers a non-intrusive incitement of the vagus nerve with no surgery. Here, the trigger is normally appended to the auricular concha by means of ear clasps and conveys electrical motivations at the subcutaneous course of the afferent auricular part of the vagus nerve. A pilot study that analyzed the utilization of VNS in 60 patients with treatment-safe burdensome issues demonstrated a noteworthy clinical improvement in 30–37% of patients and high decency. After five years, the incitement of the vagus nerve for the treatment of stubborn wretchedness was endorsed by the U.S. Nourishment and Drug Administration (FDA) (79). From that point forward, the security and adequacy of VNS in despondency have been exhibited in various observational investigations, as can be seen underneath. Conversely, there is no randomized, fake treatment control clinical preliminary that dependably exhibits energizer impacts of VNS.

The Neural Mechanism of VNS

The system by which VNS may profit patients nonresponsive to ordinary antidepressants is hazy, with further research expected to explain this. Utilitarian neuroimaging considers have affirmed that VNS adjusts the movement of numerous cortical and subcortical districts. Through immediate or roundabout anatomic associations by means of the NTS, the vagus nerve has auxiliary associations with a few mindsets directing limbic and cortical cerebrum regions. In this way, the incessant VNS for misery, PET outputs demonstrated a decrease in resting mind movement in the ventromedial prefrontal cortex (vmPFC), which activities to the amygdala and other cerebrum districts regulating feeling. VNS brings about concoction changes in monoamine digestion in these districts, conceivably bringing about energizer activity. The connection between monoamine and upper activity has been appeared by different kinds of proof. All medications that expansion monoamines—serotonin (5-HT), NE, or dopamine (DA)— in the synaptic parted have stimulant properties (86). In like manner, the consumption of monoamines initiates burdensome side effects in people who have an expanded danger of gloom.

Ceaseless VNS impacts the grouping of 5-HT, NE, and DA in the cerebrum and in the cerebrospinal liquid. In rodents, it has been demonstrated that VNS medications incite huge time-subordinate increments in basal neuronal terminating in the brainstem cores for serotonin in the dorsal raphe core. Hence, ceaseless VNS was related to expanded extracellular degrees of serotonin in the dorsal raphe.

A few lines of proof propose that NE is a synapse vital in the pathophysiology and treatment of the burdensome issue. Therefore, the exploratory consumption of NE in mind prompted an arrival of burdensome side effects after fruitful treatment with NE upper medications. The LC contains the biggest populace of noradrenergic neurons in the cerebrum and gets projections from NTS, which, thus, gets an afferent contribution from the vagus nerve. In this manner, VNS prompts an upgrade of the terminating movement of NE neurons, and therefore, an expansion in the terminating action of serotonin neurons. In this manner, VNS was appeared to build the NE fixation in the prefrontal cortex. The pharmacologic obliteration of noradrenergic neurons brought about the loss of energizer VNS impacts.

In the event of DA, it has been indicated that the transient impacts and the long haul impacts (a year) of VNS in the treatment of significant safe gloom may prompt brainstem dopaminergic enactment. DA is a catecholamine that to a huge degree, is combined in the gut and assumes an essential job in the reward framework in the cerebrum.

Further, the advantageous impacts of VNS may be applied through a monoamine-free way. Along these lines, VNS medicines may bring about unique changes of monoamine metabolites in the hippocampus, and a few examinations announced the impact of VNS on hippocampal neurogenesis. This procedure has been viewed as a key organic procedure crucial for keeping up the typical mindset.

Serotonin is additionally a significant synapse in the gut that can invigorate peristalsis and actuate sickness and heaving by enacting the vagus nerve. What's more, it is basic for the guideline of imperative capacities, for example, craving and rest, and adds to sentiments of prosperity. To 95%, it is delivered by enterochromaffin cells, a kind of neuroendocrine cell that lives close by the epithelium coating the lumen of the stomach related tract. Serotonin is discharged from enterochromaffin cells in light of mechanical or compound incitement of the gastrointestinal tract, which prompts the enactment of 5-HT3 receptors on the terminals of vagal afferents. 5-HT3 receptors are likewise present on the soma of vagal afferent neurons, including gastrointestinal vagal afferent neurons, where they can be actuated by circling 5-HT. The focal terminals of vagal afferents likewise display 5-HT3 receptors that capacity to increment glutamatergic synaptic transmission to second request neurons of the core tractus solitarius inside the brainstem. Thus, collaborations between the vagus nerve and serotonin frameworks in the gut and in the mind seem to assume a significant job in the treatment of mental conditions.

Vagus-Related Treatment of Depression

Essential Pathophysiology of Depression

Significant burdensome issue positions among the main psychological well-being reasons for the worldwide weight of sickness. With a lifetime commonness of 1.0% to 16.9% (US), the expense of sorrow represents a huge financial weight to our general public. The pathophysiology of gloom is perplexing and incorporates social, natural pressure factors, hereditary and organic procedures, for example, the overdrive of the HPA pivot, aggravation (31), and unsettling influences in monoamine neurotransmission as portrayed over. For instance, an absence of the corrosive amino tryptophan, which is an antecedent to serotonin, can instigate burdensome side effects, for example, a discouraging mindset, misery, and sadness.

The overdrive of the HPA hub is most reliably found in subjects with progressively serious (i.e., melancholic or maniacal) despondency, when the cortisol criticism inhibitory components are impeded, adding to cytokine oversecretion. It has been demonstrated that interminable presentation to raised incendiary cytokines can prompt gloom. This may be clarified by the way that cytokine overexpression prompts a decrease in serotonin levels. In accordance with that, treatment with mitigating operators can possibly decrease burdensome side effects. Inline, IBD is a significant hazard factor for mind-set and nervousness issues, and these mental conditions increment the danger of intensification of IBD.

VNS in Depression

A European multicenter study showed a beneficial outcome of VNS on burdensome manifestations in patients with treatment-safe misery. The use of VNS over a time of 3 months brought about a reaction pace of 37% and an abatement pace of 17%. Following one year of treatment, the reaction rate arrived at 53%, and the abatement rate arrived at 33%. A meta examination that contrasted the utilization of VNS with the typical treatment in discouraged patients demonstrated a reaction pace of roughly half in the intense period of the infection and a long haul reduction pace of 20% following two years of treatment. A few different investigations likewise showed an expanding long haul advantage of VNS in repetitive treatment-safe melancholy. Further, a 5-year planned observational examination which analyzed the impacts of treatment as normal and VNS as adjunctive treatment with treatment as regular just in treatment-safe wretchedness, demonstrated a superior clinical result and a higher abatement rate in the VNS gathering. This was even the situation in patients with comorbid wretchedness and uneasiness who are visit non-responders in preliminaries on stimulant medications. Note that every one of these investigations was open-mark and didn't utilize a randomized, fake treatment controlled examination plan.

Patients with sadness have raised plasma and cerebrospinal liquid convergences of proinflammatory cytokines. The advantage of VNS in wretchedness maybe because of the inhibitory activity on the generation of proinflammatory cytokines and stamped fringe increments in calming circling cytokines. Further, improvement after VNS was related to modified emission of CRH, along these lines anticipating the overdrive of the HPA hub. Modified CRH generation and emission may result from a direct stimulatory impact, transmitted from the vagus nerve through the NTS to the paraventricular core of the nerve center. At last, VNS has been appeared to restrain fringe blood generation of TNF-α which is expanded in clinical despondency.

Impact of Nutrition Depressive Symptoms

The gut microbiota is the potential key modulator of the resistant and the sensory systems. Focusing on it could prompt a more noteworthy improvement in the passionate indications of patients experiencing despondency or nervousness. There is developing proof that nourishing parts, for example, probiotics, gluten, just as medications, for example, against oxidative operators and anti-toxins, highly affect vagus nerve action through the cooperation with the gut microbiota and that this impact shifts extraordinarily between people. In reality, the creature thinks about have furnished proof that microbiota correspondence with the cerebrum includes the vagus nerve, and this cooperation can prompt intervening consequences for the mind and along these lines, conduct. For instance, Lactobacillus-species have gotten enormous consideration because of their utilization as probiotics and their wellbeing advancing properties. Bravo exhibited that ceaseless treatment of mice with Lactobacillus rhamnosus (strain JB-1) caused a decrease in pressure incited corticosterone levels and in uneasiness like and despondency like conduct. It has been demonstrated that ceaseless treatment with L. rhamnosus (JB-1) incited subordinate locale modifications in GABA(B1b) mRNA in the cerebrum with increments in cortical districts (cingulate and prelimbic) and attending decreases in articulation in the hippocampus, amygdala, and

LC. Moreover, L. rhamnosus (JB-1) diminished GABA(Aα2) mRNA articulation in the prefrontal cortex and amygdala, however, expanded GABA(Aα2) in the hippocampus, which balances the average pathogenesis of burdensome side effects: the absence of prefrontal control and overactivity of subcortical, anxiogenic cerebrum districts. Significantly, L. rhamnosus (JB-1) diminished pressure instigated corticosterone and uneasiness and gloom related conduct. This isn't amazing since changes in focal GABA receptor articulation are ensnared in the pathogenesis of uneasiness and despondency.

Controlled investigations have seen yoga-based mediations as successful in treating discouragement extending from gentle burdensome indications to significant burdensome issue (MDD) Some yoga practices can legitimately invigorate the vagus nerve, by expanding the vagal tone prompting improvement of an autonomic guideline, intellectual capacities, and disposition and stress adapting. The proposed neurophysiological systems for the accomplishment of yoga-based treatments in reducing burdensome indications recommend that yoga breathing actuates expanded vagal tone. Numerous examinations show the impacts of yogic breathing on mind work and physiologic parameters. In this way, Sudarshan Kriya Yoga (SKY), a breathing based reflective method, invigorates the vagus nerve and applies various autonomic impacts, remembering changes for a pulse, improved perception, and improved entrail work. During SKY, a grouping of breathing procedures of various frequencies, powers, lengths, and with end-inspiratory and end-expiratory holds makes shifted boosts from numerous instinctive afferents, tangible receptors, and baroreceptors. These likely impact assorted vagal strands, which thus incite physiologic changes in organs, and impact the limbic framework (140). An ongoing report indicated that even patients who didn't react to antidepressants demonstrated a critical decrease of burdensome and tension side effects contrasted with the control bunch in the wake of getting an adjunctive mediation with SKY for about two months.

Iyengar yoga has appeared to diminished burdensome side effects in subjects with wretchedness. Iyengar yoga is related to expanded HRV, supporting the speculation that yoga breathing and stances work to some extent by expanding parasympathetic tone.

Vagus-Related Treatment of PTSD

Pathophysiology of PTSD

Posttraumatic stress issue is a tension issue that can create after injury and is described by encountering nosy recollections, flashbacks, hypervigilance, bad dreams, social shirking, and social dysfunctions. It has a lifetime predominance of 8.3%, utilizing the definition for DSM-5. The indications of PTSD can be characterized into four bunches: interruption side effects, shirking conduct, intellectual and full of feeling modifications, and changes in excitement and reactivity. Individuals who experience the ill effects of PTSD will, in general, live just as under a changeless risk. They display battle and flight conduct or an unending conduct shutdown and separation, with no plausibility of arriving at a quiet state and creating positive social collaborations. After some time, these maladaptive autonomic reactions lead to the advancement of an expanded hazard for mental comorbidities, for example, dependence and cardiovascular infections.

Posttraumatic stress issue indications are incompletely interceded by the vagus nerve. There is proof for decreased parasympathetic action in PTSD, demonstrating an autonomic irregularity. The vagal control of pulse by means of the myelinated vagal strands fluctuates with the breath. Subsequently, the vagal impact on the heart can be assessed by evaluating the abundancy of cadenced variances in pulse—respiratory sinus arrhythmia (RSA). An ongoing report has shown a diminished resting RSA in veterans with PTSD (149). Further, patients with PTSD have been appeared to have lower high-recurrence pulse changeability than solid controls.

Nonstop articulation of passionate side effects to molded signs regardless of the nonattendance of extra injury is one of the numerous signs of PTSD. Conduct treatments utilized to treat PTSD depend on helping the patient to step by step lessen her/his dread of this sign after some time. In this way, presentation based treatments are viewed as the best quality level of treatment for PTSD. The objective of presentation based treatments is to supplant adapted relationship of the injury with new, progressively fitting affiliations which contend with dreadful affiliations. Studies have indicated that PTSD patients display inadequate elimination review alongside broken actuation of the dread eradication arrange. This system incorporates the vmPFC, the amygdala, and the hippocampus. It is exceptionally significant for the relevant recovery of dread recollections after eradication.

Posttraumatic stress issues side effects seriousness and auxiliary anomalies in the front hippocampus and ventromedial amygdala have been related. There is proof for expanded actuation of the amygdala in people and rodents during adapted dread. The amygdala and the vmPFC have a proportional synaptic association. In reality, under states of vulnerability and risk, the PFC can get hypoactive, prompting an inability to hinder overactivity of the amygdala with the rise of PTSD manifestations, for example, hyperarousal and re-encountering. Further, because of upsetting upgrades as dreadful faces, patients with PTSD demonstrated a higher enactment of the basolateral amygdala during oblivious face handling contrasted with sound controls just as patients with alarm issue and summed up tension issue.

The hippocampus is additionally a significant segment of the dread circuit and embroiled in the pathophysiology of PTSD. Patients with PTSD show a decreased hippocampal volume that is related to side effects seriousness. The hippocampus is a key structure in rambling memory and spatial setting encoding. Hippocampal harm prompts shortages in setting encoding in people just as rodents. The neural circuit comprising of the hippocampus, amygdala, and vmPFC is exceptionally significant for the relevant recovery of dread recollections after eradication. The impedance of hippocampal working, coming about useless setting speculation in patients with PTSD, may make patients re-experience injury-related side effects.

VNS in PTSD

Vagus nerve incitement has demonstrated guarantee as a remedial choice in treatment-safe tension issues, including PTSD. Constant VNS has been appeared to lessen nervousness in rodents and improve scores on the Hamilton Anxiety Scale in patients experiencing treatment-safe gloom. At the point when animated, the vagus nerve sends a sign to the NTS, and the NTS sends direct projections to the amygdala and the nerve center. Further, VNS builds the arrival of NE in the basolateral amygdala, just as the hippocampus and cortex. NE implantation in the amygdala brings about better termination learning. Consequently, VNS could be a decent instrument to expand termination maintenance. For instance, in rodents, termination matched with VNS treatment can prompt abatement of dread and enhancements in PTSD-like side effects. Further, VNS, combined with eradication learning, encourages the pliancy between the infralimbic average prefrontal cortex and the basolateral complex of the amygdala to encourage the annihilation of molded dread reactions (165). Moreover, VNS may likewise upgrade annihilation by restraining the action of the thoughtful sensory system. It is conceivable that a prompt VNS-initiated decrease in uneasiness adds to VNS-driven elimination by meddling with the thoughtful reaction to the CS, in this manner breaking the relationship of the CS with dread. In any case, there is a requirement for randomized controlled preliminaries to favor these perceptions.

One of the most reliable neurophysiological impacts of VNS is diminishing the hippocampal action, potentially through an upgrade of GABAergic flagging. As depicted over, the hippocampus is a vital part of the dread circuit, since it is a key structure in long-winded memory and spatial setting encoding. Diminished hippocampal movement after VNS has been accounted for in various different examinations in different conditions, for example, melancholy or schizophrenia.

Positive Influence of Nutritive Components on PTSD

Rising exploration proposes that medical probiotics may possibly diminish pressure instigated incendiary reactions, just as related side effects. An exploratory examination that researched the microbiome of patients with PTSD and injury uncovered controls uncovered a diminished presence of three microscopic organisms strains in patients with PTSD: Actinobacteria, Lentisphaerae, and Verrucomicrobia that were related with higher PTDS side effect scores. These microbes are significant for an invulnerable guideline, and their diminished wealth could have added to a dysregulation of the safe framework and advancement of PTSD indications. An examination utilizing a murine model of PTSD has exhibited that inoculation with a warmth slaughtered arrangement of the immunoregulatory bacterium Mycobacterium vaccaeinstigated an increasingly proactive social reaction to a psychosocial stressor. Studies performed in solid volunteers have indicated that the organization of various probiotics was related to improved prosperity, just as a lessening in uneasiness and mental trouble. These discoveries are altogether starter. There is a pressing requirement for well-planned, twofold visually impaired, fake treatment controlled clinical preliminaries planned for deciding the impact of bacterial enhancements and controlled changes in diet on mental side effects and psychological capacities in patients with PTSD.

Positive Influence of Meditation and Yoga on PTSD

There is clinical proof for the adequacy of care based pressure decrease (MBSR) in the treatment of PTSD. During MBSR, slow breathing and long exhalation stages lead to an expansion in parasympathetic tone. Likewise, clinical examinations have exhibited the adequacy of yoga as a restorative intercession for PTSD and separation through the downregulation of the pressure reaction. Yoga rehearses likewise diminished side effects in PSTD after catastrophic events. Yoga-responsive uneasiness issues, including PTSD, go together with low HRV and low GABA action.

Controlled examinations have seen yoga-based intercessions as effective in treating demoralization, reaching out from delicate troublesome signs to critical oppressive issues (MDD). Some yoga practices can genuinely stimulate the vagus nerve by growing the vagal tone provoking an improvement of autonomic rule, scholarly limits, and manner and stress adjusting. The proposed neurophysiological frameworks for the achievement of yoga-based medicines in diminishing troublesome signs suggest that yoga breathing impels extended vagal tone. Various assessments show the effects of yogic breathing on mind work and physiologic parameters. Along these lines, Sudarshan Kriya Yoga (SKY), a breathing based intelligent technique, empowers the vagus nerve and applies different autonomic effects, recollecting changes for the beat, improved recognition, and improved entrail work. During SKY, a gathering of breathing strategies of different frequencies, forces, lengths, and with end-inspiratory and end-expiratory holds makes moved lifts from various instinctual afferents, substantial receptors, and baroreceptors. These probable effect arranged vagal strands, which subsequently actuate physiologic changes in organs, and affect the limbic structure. A continuous report showed that even patients who didn't respond to antidepressants exhibited a basic decline of difficult and strain reactions appeared differently in relation to the control pack in the wake of getting an adjunctive intercession with SKY for around two months.

Iyengar yoga has seemed to reduced difficult reactions in subjects with wretchedness. Iyengar yoga is connected with extended HRV, supporting the hypothesis that yoga breathing and positions work somewhat by growing parasympathetic tone.

Vagus-Related Treatment of PTSD

Pathophysiology of PTSD

Posttraumatic stress issue is a strain issue that can make after damage and is portrayed by experiencing intrusive memories, flashbacks, hypervigilance, terrible dreams, social avoiding, and social dysfunctions. It has a lifetime transcendence of 8.3% using the definition for DSM-5. The signs of PTSD can be described into four bundles: interference symptoms, avoiding behavior, scholarly and brimming with feeling alterations, and changes in energy and reactivity. People who experience the evil impacts of PTSD will come by and large life similarly as under an immutable hazard. They show fight and flight direct or an unending behavior shutdown and partition, with no believability of landing at a tranquil state and making positive social joint efforts. After some time, these maladaptive autonomic responses lead to the progression of an extended risk for mental comorbidities, for instance, reliance and cardiovascular diseases.

Posttraumatic stress issue signs are deficiently intervened by the vagus nerve. There is verification for diminished parasympathetic activity in PTSD, showing an autonomic anomaly. The vagal control of heartbeat by methods for the myelinated vagal strands changes with a breath. Accordingly, the vagal effect on the heart can be surveyed by assessing the abundancy of cadenced differences in beat—respiratory sinus arrhythmia (RSA). A continuous report has demonstrated a decreased resting RSA in veterans with PTSD. Further, patients with PTSD have been seemed to have lower high-repeat beat variability than strong controls.

Relentless enunciation of enthusiastic reactions to formed signs paying little respect to the nonattendance of additional damage is one of the various indications of PTSD. Direct medications used to treat PTSD rely upon helping the patient to bit by bit reduce her/his fear of this sign after some time. Along these lines, introduction based medicines are seen as the best quality degree of treatment for PTSD The target of introduction based medicines is to displace adjusted relationship of the damage with new, dynamically fitting affiliations which battle with repulsive affiliations. Studies have demonstrated that PTSD patients show a deficient disposal survey close by broken incitation of the fear of annihilation orchestrate. This framework joins the vmPFC, the amygdala, and the hippocampus. It is uncommonly huge for the significant recuperation of fear memories after annihilation.

Posttraumatic stress issue reaction earnestness and assistant irregularities in the front hippocampus and ventromedial amygdala have been connected. There is confirmation for extended activation of the amygdala in individuals and rodents during adjusted fear. The amygdala and the vmPFC have relative synaptic affiliations. In all actuality, under conditions of defenselessness and hazard, the PFC can get hypoactive, provoking a failure to prevent overactivity of the amygdala with the ascent of PTSD appearances, for instance, hyperarousal and re-experiencing. Further, in light of upsetting redesigns as terrifying faces, patients with PTSD exhibited a higher authorization of the basolateral amygdala during unmindful face taking care of stood out from sound controls similarly as patients with an alert issue and summarized pressure issue.

The hippocampus is furthermore a noteworthy fragment of the fear circuit and entangled in the pathophysiology of PTSD. Patients with PTSD show a diminished hippocampal volume that is connected with reaction earnestness. The hippocampus is a key structure in meandering memory and spatial setting encoding aimlessly. Hippocampal hurt prompts deficiencies in setting encoding in individuals similarly as rodents. The neural circuit containing the hippocampus, amygdala, and vmPFC is incredibly noteworthy for the important recuperation of fear memories after annihilation (154). The impedance of hippocampal working, coming about pointless setting theory in patients with PTSD, may make patients re-experience damage related symptoms.

VNS in PTSD

Vagus nerve actuation has shown to ensure as a medicinal decision in the treatment-safe strain issue, including PTSD. Steady VNS has been seemed to diminish apprehension in rodents and improve scores on the Hamilton Anxiety Scale in patients encountering treatment-safe misery. Exactly when enlivened, the vagus nerve sends the sign to the NTS, and the NTS sends direct projections to the amygdala and the operational hub. Further, VNS fabricates the appearance of NE in the basolateral amygdala, similarly to the hippocampus and cortex. NE implantation in the amygdala realizes better end learning. Thusly, VNS could be a fair instrument to extend end upkeep. For example, in rodents, end coordinated with VNS treatment can provoke the reduction of fear and improvements in PTSD-like reactions. Further, VNS joined with destruction learning supports the malleability between the infralimbic normal prefrontal cortex and the basolateral complex of the amygdala to empower the demolition of shaped fear responses. Additionally, VNS may similarly update demolition by limiting the activity of the keen tactile framework. It is possible that a brief VNS-started decline in uneasiness adds to VNS-driven disposal by interfering with the mindful response to the CS, as such breaking the relationship of the CS with fear. Regardless, there is a prerequisite for randomized controlled starters to support these discernments.

One of the most dependable neurophysiological effects of VNS is reducing the hippocampal activity, a conceivably thorough overhaul of GABAergic hailing. As delineated over, the hippocampus is a crucial piece of the fear circuit, since it is a key structure in verbose memory and spatial setting encoding. Reduced hippocampal development after VNS has been represented in various different assessments in various conditions, for instance, despairing or schizophrenia.

Positive Influence of Nutritive Components on PTSD

Rising investigation suggests that probiotics may lessen pressure incited flammable responses, similarly as related reactions. An exploratory assessment that examined the microbiome of patients with PTSD and damage revealed controls uncovered a reduced nearness of three tiny living beings strains in patients with PTSD: Actinobacteria, Lentisphaerae, and Verrucomicrobia that were connected with higher PTSD symptom scores. These microorganisms are huge for a safe rule, and their decreased riches could have added to a dysregulation of the protected structure and headway of PTSD signs. An assessment using a murine model of PTSD has shown that vaccination with a glow butchered course of action of the immunoregulatory bacterium Mycobacterium vaccae (NCTC 11659) incited an undeniably proactive social response to a psychosocial stressor. Studies performed in strong volunteers have shown that the association of different probiotics was connected with improved success, similarly as a decreasing in a difficult situation (174, These revelations are through and through the starter. There is a squeezing necessity for well-arranged, twofold outwardly disabled, counterfeit treatment controlled clinical fundamentals got ready for choosing the effect of bacterial improvements and controlled changes in diet on mental reactions and mental limits in patients with PTSD.

Positive Influence of Meditation and Yoga on PTSD

There is clinical verification for the ampleness of care based weight decline (MBSR) in the treatment of PTSD.

The association between the gut and the cerebrum depends on an intricate framework that incorporates neural as well as endocrine, resistant, and humoral connections.

The vagus nerve is a fundamental piece of the cerebrum gut pivot and assumes a significant job in the adjustment of irritation, the upkeep of intestinal homeostasis, and the guideline of nourishment admission, satiety, and vitality homeostasis. A communication among nourishment and the vagus nerve is notable, and vagal tone can impact nourishment admission and weight gain.

Besides, the vagus nerve assumes a significant job in the pathogenesis of mental issues, the weight just as different pressure incited and fiery sicknesses.

Vagus nerve incitement and a few reflection strategies exhibit that regulating the vagus nerve has a helpful impact, principally because of its unwinding and mitigating properties.

Eradication matched with VNS is faster than termination combined with hoax incitement. As it is now affirmed by the Federal FDA for despondency and seizure avoidance, VNS is a promptly accessible and promising subordinate to presentation treatment for the treatment of extreme nervousness issues.

Vagus nerve incitement is a compelling anticonvulsant gadget and has appeared in observational investigations energizer impacts in interminable treatment-safe wretchedness. Since the vagus nerve sends data to mind districts is significant in the pressure reaction (LC, orbitofrontal cortex, insula, hippocampus, and amygdala), this pathway may be engaged with seeing or showing different physical and psychological side effects that portray pressure-related issue.

Psychotropic medications, for example, serotonin reuptake inhibitors, have impacts on both the mind and the gastrointestinal tract and thusly ought to be comprehended as modulators of the cerebrum gut hub.

Research exploring the collaboration between nutritive elements, substantial components, for example, pulse, mental and pharmacological medications, and vagal action can possibly prompt integrative treatment alternatives that join VNS, dietary methodologies, drugs, and mental intercessions, for example, care based methodologies, which can be custom fitted to the necessities of the individual patient.

Chapter Three: How is it composed, and how does it work?

The vagus nerve is the longest nerve of the autonomic sensory system and is one of the most significant nerves in the body. The vagus nerve manages numerous basic parts of human physiology, including the pulse, circulatory strain, perspiring, assimilation, and in any event, talking. Thus, restorative science has since a long time ago looked for methods for regulating the capacity of the vagus nerve.

Life structures of the Vagus Nerve

The vagus nerve (otherwise called the tenth cranial nerve or CN X) is an exceptionally long nerve that starts in the cerebrum stem and reaches out down through the neck and into the chest and mid-region. On the off chance that conveys both engine and tactile data, and it supplies innervation to the heart, significant veins, aviation routes, lungs, throat, stomach, and digestive organs.

While there are really two vagus nerves (the left and the right), specialists normally allude to them together as "the vagus nerve." The vagus nerve helps control a few muscles of the throat and of the voicebox. It assumes a significant job in controlling the pulse and keeping the gastrointestinal tract in working request. The vagus nerves likewise convey tactile data from the inside organs back to the mind.

The capacity of the Vagus Nerve

Maybe the best importance of the vagus nerve is that it is the body's significant parasympathetic nerve, providing parasympathetic strands to all the significant organs of the head, neck, chest, and guts. The vagus nerve is answerable for the muffle reflex (and the hack reflex when the ear waterway is invigorated), easing back the pulse, controlling perspiring, managing circulatory strain, animating peristalsis of the gastrointestinal tract, and controlling vascular tone.

The Vasovagal Reflex

Unexpected incitement of a vagus nerve can create what is known as a "vasovagal reflex," which comprises of an abrupt drop in pulse and an easing back of the pulse. This reflex can be activated by gastrointestinal sickness or in light of torment, dread, or abrupt pressure. A few people are especially inclined to the vasovagal reflex, and their circulatory strain and pulse changes can cause loss of cognizance — a condition called "vasovagal syncope."

Inordinate enactment of the vagus nerve is likewise found in certain ailments, particularly the dysautonomias.

Invigorating the vagus nerve can have restorative impacts, (for example, halting scenes of supraventricular tachycardia (SVT) or hiccups), and can assist specialists with diagnosing specific sorts of heart mumbles. Vagal incitement can be accomplished effectively by utilizing the Valsalva move.

The Vagus Nerve and the Heart

The correct vagus nerve supplies the sinus hub, and its incitement can create sinus bradycardia. The left vagus nerve supplies the AV hub, and its incitement can deliver a type of heart square. It is by creating transient heart obstruct that the Valsalva move can end numerous sorts of SVT.

The Vagus Nerve in Medical Therapy

Since the vagus nerve has such a significant number of significant capacities, therapeutic science has been keen on decades in utilizing vagus nerve incitement, or vagus nerve obstructing, in restorative treatment.

For a considerable length of time, the vagotomy system (cutting the vagus nerve) was a backbone of treatment for peptic ulcer illness, since this was a method for decreasing the measure of peptic corrosive being delivered by the stomach. Nonetheless, the vagotomy had a few unfavorable impacts, and with the accessibility of progressively viable treatment has now become significantly less ordinarily utilized.

Today, there is extraordinary enthusiasm for utilizing electronic triggers (basically, altered pacemakers) to constantly invigorate the vagus nerve trying to treat different medicinal issues. Such gadgets (alluded to conventionally as vagus nerve invigorating gadgets, or VNS gadgets) have been utilized effectively to treat individuals with extreme epilepsy that is recalcitrant to sedate treatment. VNS treatment is additionally now and again used to treat unmanageable despondency.

Since when you have a sled, everything resembles a nail, organizations that make VNS gadgets are researching their use in a few different conditions including hypertension, headaches, tinnitus, fibromyalgia, and weight reduction.

There is to be a sure guarantee in such utilization of VNS. Be that as it may, the genuine capability of VNS will develop once the promotion is supplanted by firm clinical proof.

Why the Vagus Nerve is so Important

After my significant other died, sometime in the past, my pressure was so high that I was having a go at everything conceivable to decrease it-- -- from dietary solutions for vitality mending. In a minute that I'll always remember, a vitality healer that I was seeing let me know, "your focal sensory system is seared, and I'm truly stressed over you."

Presently this may appear to be somewhat "out there" and charm to a few, however, this lady had helped me mend from such huge numbers of the issues I was managing, and for her to disclose to me that she was worried about a piece of my body that I had generally been totally ignorant of was a major AHA minute for me. I had no clue that there was a nerve that was at the base of my focal sensory system issues, and still today, I locate that a couple of individuals realize how to quiet it or expertise to invigorate it appropriately.

The vagus nerve (articulated Vegas) controls such a large number of significant capacities in your body from your breathing to your pulse, and when it's appropriately animated, it can serve basically as a "hack" to your legitimate wellbeing. Issues with your focal sensory system regularly go unnoticed, in light of the fact that you probably won't have the option to feel them straightforwardly, or they may show themselves in various manners, as through your gut or your cerebrum. That is the reason this nerve is so significant – by discovering approaches to keep it working appropriately; you can jump over your wellbeing and fix any issues even before they begin to show.

For what reason is the vagus nerve so significant?

The vagus nerve is likely one of the most little-known yet, in addition, one of the most significant nerves in your body. It assumes a job in such a significant number of indispensable capacities in our body, from the "rest and overviews" duties of our parasympathetic sensory system to the "battle or flight" reaction directed by our thoughtful sensory system. The nerve ranges from the mind through the neck and stomach area, right to the colon– – which enables it to send tactile data all through the body.

Not exclusively is this nerve attached to our body's standard day by day works like pulse, breathing, and preparing recollections. However, it additionally assumes a fundamental job in one of the present most discussed wellbeing subjects – the gut. Basically, the vagus nerve can detect the microbiota in your gut and send tangible signs and data to the focal sensory system, where the body at that point inspires an appropriate reaction. So what precisely does that mean? That your mind and gut truly are associated, and the vagus nerve fills in as the primary concern of contact between the two. With the goal, that's the reason, when you're focused on, you may likewise have a disturbed stomach or a few issues in the washroom – stress represses the vagus nerve, which can lose the gastrointestinal framework and lead to issues like IBS and IBD (fiery inside illness). In any case, when the vagus nerve is animated, it's calming properties can make genuinely necessary homeostasis in the gut.

How might you bolster your vagus nerve?

At the point when your vagus nerve is animated and working appropriately, it can do stunning things for your body. Studies have demonstrated that animating the vagus nerve can have upper, mitigating, gut-boosting, mind boosting benefits... thus some more! In any case, how would you benefit from the wellbeing supports that may originate from an appropriately invigorated vagus nerve? Here is a portion of the ways:

Profound breathing – A recent report demonstrated that members who rehearsed moderate, the stomach had upgraded vagal nerve action. Have a go at setting down in an agreeable spot with a hand on your mid-region. Take in through your nose and hold it for a couple of moments, feeling the air fill your mid-region and gradually discharge through your mouth. Rehash these means for in any event 10 minutes of the day.

Irregular fasting – More than only an eating routine pattern, it considers showing that discontinuous fasting can animate the vagus nerve.

Taking probiotics – We previously talked about how we can thank the vagus nerve for the one of a kind gut-mind association, however certain bacterial and wholesome upgrades (like probiotics, for instance) can improve the nerve and the sign it sends.

Show sympathy – Obviously, this is something we ought to do constantly, however being pleasant and sympathetic to others can likewise have some close to home advantages, particularly for this significant nerve. Not exclusively can indicating sympathy can invigorate the vagus nerve, by method for the mind, yet in addition, those with a functioning and animated vagus nerve are bound to be unselfish and empathetic individuals – it's a cycle that will leave you feeling incredible about yourself as well as other people!

Practice yoga – An ordinary yoga practice can animate your vagus nerve and upgrade the yield of your parasympathetic framework, which can prompt helped disposition, vitality, and heart work.

Chapter Four: The functions of the vagus nerve

Anatomical Course

The vagus nerve has the longest course of all the cranial nerves, reaching out from the head to the mid-region. Its name is gotten from the Latin 'idea' – which means meandering. It is, in some cases, alluded to as the meandering nerve.

In the Head

The vagus nerve starts from the medulla of the brainstem. It leaves the noggin by means of the jugular foramen, with the glossopharyngeal and extra nerves (CN IX and XI separately).

Inside the head, the auricular branch emerges — this provision sensation to the back piece of the outer sound-related channel and outside the ear.

In the Neck

In the neck, the vagus nerve goes into the carotid sheath, voyaging poorly with the inner jugular vein and regular carotid conduit. At the base of the neck, the privilege and left nerves have varying pathways:

The correct vagus nerve passes front to the subclavian conduit and back to the sternoclavicular joint, entering the thorax.

The left vagus nerve passes poorly between the left regular carotid and left subclavian supply routes, back to the sternoclavicular joint, entering the thorax.

A few branches emerge in the neck:

- Pharyngeal branches – Provides engine innervation to most of the muscles of the pharynx and delicate sense of taste.
- Predominant laryngeal nerve – Splits into inside and outside branches. The outer laryngeal nerve innervates the cricothyroid muscle of the larynx. The interior laryngeal gives tactile innervation to the

laryngopharynx and predominant piece of the larynx.

- Intermittent laryngeal nerve (right side just) – Hooks underneath the privilege subclavian supply route, at that point, climbs towards the larynx. It innervates most of the inborn muscles of the larynx.

In the Thorax

In the thorax, the correct vagus nerve frames the back vagal trunk, and the left structures the foremost vagal trunk. Branches from the vagal trunks add to the development of the oesophageal plexus, which innervates the smooth muscle of the throat.

Two different branches emerge in the thorax:

- Left repetitive laryngeal nerve – it snares under the curve of the aorta, climbing to innervate most of the inherent muscles of the larynx.
- Cardiovascular branches – these innervate direct pulse and give instinctive sensation to the organ.

The vagal trunks enter the belly by means of the oesophageal break, an opening in the stomach.

In the Abdomen

In the belly, the vagal trunks end by isolating into branches that supply the throat, stomach, and the little and enormous entrail (up to the splenic flexure).

Tactile Functions

There are physical and instinctive parts to the tangible capacity of the vagus nerve.

Physical alludes to sensation from the skin and muscles. This is given by the auricular nerve, which innervates the skin of the back piece of the outer sound-related channel and outside the ear.

Viscera sensation is from the organs of the body. The vagus nerve innervates:

- Laryngopharynx – by means of the inside laryngeal nerve.
- Prevalent part of the larynx (above vocal folds) – by means of the inferior laryngeal nerve.

- Heart – by means of cardiovascular parts of the vagus nerve.
- Gastrointestinal tract (up to the splenic flexure) – by means of the terminal parts of the vagus nerve.

Uncommon Sensory Functions

The vagus nerve has a minor job in taste sensation. It conveys afferent filaments from the foundation of the tongue and epiglottis.

The vagus nerve speaks to the principle segment of the parasympathetic sensory system, which supervises a huge range of real essential capacities, including control of temperament, insusceptible reaction, assimilation, and pulse. It sets up one of the associations between the cerebrum and the gastrointestinal tract and sends data about the condition of the internal organs to the mind by means of afferent filaments. In this audit, we examine different elements of the vagus nerve which make it an appealing objective in treating mental and gastrointestinal issues. There is primer proof that vagus nerve incitement is a promising extra treatment for treatment-headstrong melancholy, posttraumatic stress issue, and incendiary inside sickness. Medications that focus on the vagus nerve increment the vagal tone and restrain cytokine generation. Both are significant components of flexibility. The incitement of vagal afferent filaments in the gut impacts monoaminergic mind frameworks in the cerebrum stem that assume critical jobs in major mental conditions, for example, state of mind and tension issue. Inline, there is primer proof for gut microscopic organisms to have a gainful impact on the state of mind and uneasiness, somewhat by influencing the action of the vagus nerve. Since the vagal tone is corresponded with the ability to control pressure reactions and can be affected by breathing, its expansion through contemplation and yoga likely adds to the strength and the moderation of state of mind and tension manifestations.

The bidirectional correspondence between the mind and the gastrointestinal tract, the purported "cerebrum gut hub," depends on an unpredictable framework, including the vagus nerve, yet in addition thoughtful (e.g., by means of the prevertebral ganglia), endocrine, safe, and humoral connections just as the impact of gut microbiota so as to direct gastrointestinal homeostasis and to associate enthusiastic and psychological zones of the cerebrum with gut capacities. The ENS delivers in excess of 30 synapses and has a larger number of neurons than the spine. Hormones and peptides that the ENS discharges into the blood dissemination cross the blood–mind obstruction (e.g., ghrelin) and can act synergistically with the vagus nerve, for instance, to direct nourishment admission and craving. The mind-gut pivot is getting progressively significant as a helpful objective for gastrointestinal and mental issues, for example, fiery inside malady (IBD), gloom, and posttraumatic stress issue (PTSD). The gut is a significant control focal point of the resistant framework, and the vagus nerve has immunomodulatory properties. Therefore, this nerve assumes significant jobs in the connection between the gut, the cerebrum, and irritation. There are new treatment choices for regulating the cerebrum gut hub, for instance, vagus nerve incitement (VNS) and contemplation methods. These medicines have been demonstrated to be valuable in state of mind and tension issue, yet additionally in different conditions related to expanded aggravation (10). Specifically, gut-coordinated hypnotherapy was demonstrated to be viable in both, crabby inside disorder and IBD. At last, the vagus nerve likewise speaks to a significant connection among sustenance and mental, neurological and fiery infections.

The benefits of Vagus Nerve By Kelly

Kelly Owens recollects the first occasion when she felt wiped out. As a 13-year-old who cherished everything from ball and field hockey to theater, she was a heap of vitality. In this way, when she bent her lower leg during a network theater practice for "The Music Man," she was crushed as it expand up.

In spite of confirmations that it was simply minor damage, it never showed signs of improvement. In the long run, her primary care physician expelled 10 milliliters of liquid from her lower leg just to have it return the exceptionally same night. Half a month later, she began encountering gastrointestinal trouble so serious she had to leave class at regular intervals to go to the restroom.

"I felt confounded," Kelly said. "To go from being a functioning, athletic child, to out of the blue having my body appear to be at war with me at that youthful of age, felt peculiar. Everything abruptly felt remote and out of my control."

The conclusion came before long: Crohn's malady — an aggravation of the gastrointestinal track — with signs of incendiary joint inflammation.

Kelly battled for the following 16 years to oversee side effects and battle Crohn's. The joint pain spread to each other joint in her body, as far as possible up to her jaw. She experienced colitis and other Crohn's side effects, similar to ulcers on her legs. She attempted each possible medication accessible to squelch her indications and calm the irritation.

"I've been on each biologic, DMARD, and immunosuppressant under the sun accessible for Crohn's ailment," said Kelly. "None of them worked for a really long time, if by any means," she said. "My body constantly developed antibodies against everything, and in addition, these prescriptions made me feel like an atomic power plant. For a long time, the main thing that held me over were steroids."

In any case, long haul steroids have symptoms as well. By 25, Kelly was determined to have osteoporosis brought about by the constant utilization of this drug, just as malabsorption because of the colitis.

That equivalent year, Owens was living in Hawaii and instructing English. "I'd get back home from work, prop my knees up on cushions, and ice my legs while evaluating and exercise arranging. At that point, I'd do it once more the following day... until I couldn't any longer," she said.

While perusing the Huffington Post, she found a meeting of Kevin J. Tracey, a neurosurgeon and the CEO of the Feinstein Institute for Medical Research, talking about the bioelectronic drugs. His examination demonstrated how the little destroys of power to the vagus nerve could stop the over-creation of incendiary cytokines. "As I watched him clarify this in the meeting," Kelly stated, "I realized this gadget would in the long run completely change me. I found his email and revealed to him my story." At that point in time, in 2014, Tracey's vagus incitement look into was being taken a stab at rheumatoid joint inflammation patients. In the meantime, Kelly's manifestations intensified, so a lot of that she needed to quit educating.

It wasn't until mid-2017 when her primary care physicians educated her; there were no more drugs left to attempt that Kelly reached Tracey once more. SetPoint Medical had quite recently begun a clinical preliminary utilizing vagus nerve incitement for Crohn's malady.

By July, Owens experienced an exploratory strategy embedding a battery-sized gadget into her chest to convey modest quantities of electrical incitement to her vagus nerve. The outcome has been groundbreaking.

"I simply don't have side effects any longer," Kelly says. "Dislike manifestations creep back up around evening time or toward the beginning of the day or whenever in the middle of — and my body finds a sense of contentment. For a lady that couldn't stroll for in excess of a couple of moments without expecting to rest and now and then required a wheelchair, I currently wind up going on climbs that can keep going for miles, running on the treadmill, and rediscovering what my body is able to do."

Vagus nerve incitement (VNS) worked for Owens since it hosed the incendiary markers causing her Crohn's infection and joint pain. For Owens, VNS focuses on her spleen to lessen the generation of genius fiery cytokines. Be that as it may, VNS isn't just used to treat fiery conditions, partially on the grounds that the vagus nerve impacts such a significant number of parts of the body. As the body's longest cranial nerve, the vagus nerve has tangible and engine filaments running from the brainstem through different organs, including the heart, lungs, stomach, and digestive organs, finishing off with the colon.

In the course of the most recent 30 years, VNS has been utilized to treat different maladies, including treatment-safe discouragement, treatment-safe epilepsy, incessant headaches, and group cerebral pains. VNS gadgets are ordinarily embedded, like Kelly's, however, as of late, non-intrusive adaptations of VNS, which can be applied through your ear, are likewise being investigated.

Dr. Matthew Leonard, Assistant Professor of Neurological Surgery in the Weill Institute for Neurosciences at the University of California, San Francisco, has been investigating non-intrusive VNS's utilization in language learning. In one of Leonard's ongoing investigations, non-intrusive VNS had the option to upgrade individuals' capacity to gain proficiency with an outstanding phonetic test: Mandarin tones.

Be that as it may, it's as yet hazy how comparative non-intrusive VNS is to an embedded VNS gadget, which is the reason Leonard's group is as of now attempting to look at the two. "We record neural movement straightforwardly from the human mind in patients with epilepsy, some of whom additionally as of now have embedded cervical VNS gadgets, and who volunteer to wear our ear gadget for a couple of moments," said Leonard. This enables these analysts to check whether the incitement in mind is comparable between these intrusive and non-obtrusive methodologies.

It's not in any case pretty much the sort of gadget — there are different elements, similar to the quality of the incitement, how it's applied, and even the anode materials that can assume a job in VNS. As indicated by Leonard, "the field is in an exploratory stage at the present time, as we research moves toward that can connect with this misleadingly basic nerve in a wide cluster of utilizations."

Regular Ways to Stimulate the Vagus Nerve

Obviously, vagus nerve incitement is significant for ideal wellbeing. There is an FDA controlled gadget that you can have embedded in the body. It sends electrical driving forces to animate the vagus nerve. Be that as it may, there are different methods for animating the vagus nerve without medical procedure, gadgets, or symptoms.

The cold treatment has numerous advantages from quicker recuperation from exercise to improved resistant capacity. Intense cold presentation additionally enacts the vagus nerve and cholinergic neurons and nitrergic neurons through vagus nerve pathways, as per a recent report. This implies cold introduction can likewise expand parasympathetic movement through the vagus nerve, bringing down the thoughtful (battle or flight) reaction.

Profound Breathing

It's notable that profound, slow breathing can help actuate unwinding. As referenced before, vagal incitement can cause unwinding; however, the inverse is additionally valid. Unwinding can invigorate the vagal nerve. So prompting unwinding through profound breathing can help improve vagal tone. This will at that point, make it simpler to get into a casual state later on!

Singing, Humming, Gargling

Singing and murmuring might be unwinding without anyone else, yet there's a physiological explanation behind it. The vagus nerve is joined to the vocal strings. Research distributed in Frontiers in Psychology shows that singing, murmuring, and in any event, swishing can help enact it. Biting additionally animates vagus nerve movement (and the parasympathetic framework that enacts assimilation, which bodes well!). This implies biting gum, while it might have its drawbacks, additionally animates the vagus nerve.

Irregular Fasting

Be that as it may, it turns out these medical advantages might be identified with discontinuous fasting's capacity to invigorate the vagus nerve and improve vagal tone. A recent report found that fasting is a physiological activator of the vagus nerve. Wave vibration has been intensely contemplated by mainstream researchers for its medical advantages. This treatment includes remaining on a swaying plate that produces low-level vibrations. These vibrations, at that point, make positive worry all through the body (like the sort of stress made by work out). This pressure initiates the vagal nerve among different pieces of the body.

Exercise

Exercise is a significant piece of a solid way of life. Be that as it may, it would seem that it might likewise be useful in invigorating the vagus nerve. This could be the explanation that activity causes us to unwind. One 2010 examination found that mellow exercise invigorated gastric exhausting and improved processing. They found this happened in view of vagal incitement.

Backrub

The research proposes that back rub can be valuable in invigorating the vagus nerve. In one 2012 examination, untimely babies who were kneaded had a more noteworthy weight increase because of vagal action. This is one explanation we attempt to utilize an assortment of back rub systems and devices at home.

Vagus Nerve as a Link between the Central and ENS

The association between the CNS and the ENS likewise alluded to as the mind-gut pivot, empowers the bidirectional association between the cerebrum and the gastrointestinal tract. It is liable for observing the physiological homeostasis and associating the enthusiastic and intellectual regions of the mind with fringe intestinal capacities, for example, safe actuation, intestinal porousness, enteric reflex, and enteroendocrine flagging. This mind-gut pivot, incorporates the cerebrum, the spinal rope, the autonomic sensory system (thoughtful, parasympathetic, and ENS), and the hypothalamic-pituitary-adrenal (HPA) hub. The vagal efferents send the sign "down" from mind to gut through efferent filaments, which represent 10–20% of everything being equal and the vagal afferents "up" from the intestinal divider to the cerebrum representing 80–90% all things considered.

The vagus nerve fills in as the body's superhighway, conveying data between the mind and the inside organs and controlling the body's reaction in the midst of rest and unwinding. The enormous nerve begins in mind and branches out in various ways to the neck and middle, where it's liable for activities, for example, conveying tactile data from the skin of the ear, controlling the muscles that you use to swallow and talk and impacting your safe framework.

The vagus is the tenth of 12 cranial nerves that expand straightforwardly from the mind, as indicated by the Encyclopedia Britannica. In spite of the fact that we allude to the vagus nerve as particular, it's really a couple of nerves that rise up out of the left and right half of the medulla oblongata bit of the cerebrum stem. The nerve gets its name from the Latin word for meandering, as indicated by Merriam-Webster, which is suitable, as the vagus nerve is the biggest and most broadly spreading cranial nerve.

By meandering and expanding all through the body, the vagus nerve gives the essential control to the sensory system's parasympathetic division: the rest-and-condensation contradiction to the thoughtful sensory system's battle or-flight reaction. At the point when the body isn't under pressure, the vagus nerve sends directions that moderate heart and breathing rates and increment processing. In the midst of stress, control movements to the thoughtful framework, which delivers the contrary impact.

The vagus nerve additionally conveys tangible signs from inward organs back to the mind, empowering the cerebrum to monitor the organs' activities.

The mind-gut pivot

Huge divisions of the vagus nerve reach out to the stomach related framework. About 10% to 20% of the vagus nerve cells that interface with the stomach related framework sends directions from the cerebrum to control muscles that move nourishment through the gut, as per the reading material "Nerves and Nerve Injuries Volume 1" (Academic Press, 2015). The development of those muscles is then constrained by a different sensory system installed inside the dividers of the stomach related framework.

The staying 80% to 90% of the neurons convey tactile data from the stomach and digestion tracts to the mind. This correspondence line between the cerebrum and the gastrointestinal tract is known as the mind-gut hub, and it keeps the cerebrum educated about the status of muscle withdrawal, the speed of nourishment entry through the gut, and sentiments of craving or satiety. A recent report distributed in the Journal of Internal Medicine found that the vagus nerve is so intently laced with the stomach related framework that incitement of the nerve can improve crabby inside disorder.

In late decades, numerous analysts have discovered that this mind-gut hub has another partner — the microbes that live inside the digestion tracts. This microbiome speaks with the cerebrum through the vagus nerve, influencing nourishment to allow as well as state of mind and irritation reaction, as indicated by a 2014 audit distributed in the diary Advances in Experimental Medicine and Biology. A significant part of the current research includes explores different avenues regarding mice and rodents as opposed to people. In any case, the outcomes are striking and show that adjustments in the microbiome may cause changes in the mind.

Vagus nerve incitement as a restorative treatment

The incitement of the vagus nerve has been successful in treating instances of epilepsy that don't react to the medicine. Specialists place a terminal around the correct part of the vagus nerve in the neck, with a battery embedded underneath the collarbone. The terminal gives standard incitement to the nerve, which diminishes, or in uncommon cases counteracts, the over the top cerebrum action that causes seizures, as indicated by the Epilepsy Foundation. Europe has endorsed a vagus nerve trigger that doesn't require careful implantation, as per the Mayo Clinic.

Research has likewise indicated that vagus nerve incitement could be powerful for treating mental conditions that don't react to prescription. The FDA has endorsed vagus nerve incitement for treatment-safe sadness and for bunch migraines. A recent report distributed in the diary Brain Stimulation found that vagus nerve incitement brought about an improvement in manifestations for patients with treatment-safe nervousness issues, for example, over the top impulsive issue, alarm issue, and post-horrible pressure issue.

All the more as of late, analysts have been exploring the vagus nerve's job in treating the constant incendiary issues, for example, sepsis, lung damage, rheumatoid joint pain (RA), and diabetes, as indicated by a 2018 survey in the Journal of Inflammation Research. Since the vagus nerve impacts the safe framework, harm to the nerve may have a job in the immune system and different issues.

Harm to the vagus nerve

Researchers have since quite a while ago referred to that constant conditions, for example, liquor abuse and diabetes can harm nerves, including the vagus nerve, despite the fact that why this harm happens isn't surely known. Individuals with insulin-subordinate diabetes may create neuropathy in numerous nerves. On the off chance that the vagus nerve is harmed, queasiness, swelling, the runs, and gastroparesis (in which the stomach exhausts too gradually) may result. Lamentably, diabetic neuropathy can't be turned around, as indicated by the Mayo Clinic.

On the off chance that the vagus nerve gets harmed by physical injury or the development of a tumor, it might cause stomach related manifestations, or dryness, loss of motion of the vocal lines and eased back pulse. There have been a few instances of individuals whose vagus nerve harm was little enough that the nerve had the option to recover after the evacuation of a tumor, including a 2011 case nitty-gritty in the diary Neurology.

The vagus nerve and blacking out

At the point when somebody blacks out from heat presentation, representing quite a while or from something astounding, for example, seeing blood, the vagus nerve is halfway to a fault. This event, called vasovagal syncope, happens when the thoughtful division widens veins in the legs, and the vagus nerve goes overboard, causing a noteworthy and prompt lessening in pulse. Blood pools in the legs, pulse drops, and without enough bloodstream to the mind, the individual loses awareness quickly. Except if an individual swoon every now and again, vasovagal syncope doesn't require treatment.

It keeps up your pulse and makes you sweat. It encourages you to talk and makes you upchuck. It's your vagus nerve, and it's the data expressway that associates your mind with organs all through the body.

Vagus is Latin for "meandering." And this nerve certainly realizes how to meander aimlessly. It extends from the cerebrum right down the middle. En route, it contacts key organs, for example, the heart and stomach. This gives the vagus authority over an enormous scope of real capacities.

A large portion of the cranial (KRAY-nee-ul) nerves — 12 enormous nerves that leave the base of the mind — arrive at just a couple of bits of the body. They may control vision, hearing, or the vibe of a solitary finger against your cheek. Be that as it may, the vagus — number 10 out of those 12 nerves — assumes many jobs. What's more, the greater part of them are capacities you never deliberately think about, from the inclination inside your ear to the muscles that help you talk.

The vagus starts in the medulla oblongata (Meh-DU-lah (Ah-blon-GAH-tah). It's the most reduced piece of the mind and sits simply above where the cerebrum converges into the spinal rope. The vagus is really two huge nerves — long filaments made out of numerous littler cells that send data around the body. One develops on the correct side of the medulla, another on the left. However, the vast majority allude to both the privilege and left simultaneously when they talk about "the vagus."

From the medulla, the vagus climbs, down and around the body. For example, it comes up to touch within the ear. Further down, the nerve helps control the muscles of the larynx. That is the piece of the throat containing the vocal lines. From the back of the throat as far as possible of the digestive organ, portions of the nerve wrap delicately around all of these cylinders and organs. It additionally contacts the bladder and sticks a sensitive finger into the heart.

Resting and processing

This present nerve's job is near as fluctuated as its goals. How about we start at the top.

In the ear, it forms the feeling of touch, filling somebody in as to whether there's something inside their ear. In the throat, the vagus controls the muscles of the vocal strings. This enables individuals to talk. It additionally controls the developments of the back of the throat and is liable for the pharyngeal reflex (FAIR-en-GEE-ul REE-flex). Otherwise called the stifler reflex, it can make somebody upchuck. All the more regularly, this reflex essentially helps shield objects from getting trapped in the throat where they could make somebody gag.

Further down, the vagus nerve folds over the stomach related tract, including the throat (Ee-SOF-uh-guys), stomach, and the huge and small digestive organs. The vagus controls peristalsis (Pair-ih-STAHL-sister) — the wavelike withdrawal of muscles that move nourishment through the gut.

More often than not, it is barely noticeable your vagus. It's an enormous piece of what's known as the parasympathetic sensory system. That is a long haul to depict that piece of the sensory system that controls what occurs without our intuition about it. It enables the body to do things that it's procrastinated on for when it's casual, for example, processing nourishment, recreating, or peeing.

At the point when turned on, the vagus nerve can slow the heart's thumping and lower circulatory strain. The nerve additionally ventures into the lungs, where it controls how quick you relax. The vagus even controls the smooth muscle that agreements the bladder when you pee. As noted before, it directs perspiring, as well.

This nerve can even make individuals blackout. Here are the means by which: When somebody is amazingly focused on, the vagus nerve can get overstimulated as it attempts to cut down pulse and circulatory strain. This may make somebody's pulse hinder excessively. A circulatory strain may now fall. Under these conditions, too little blood arrives at the head — making somebody blackout. This is called vasovagal syncope (Vay-zoh-VAY-gul SING-kuh-pee).

The vagus is anything but a single direction road. It's extremely progressively like a two-way, six-path superhighway. This nerve sends a flag out of the cerebrum; at that point gets criticism from stations all through the body. Those cell tips return to the mind and enable it to monitor every organ the vagus contacts.

Data from the body not exclusively can change how the mind controls the vagus, yet can likewise influence the cerebrum itself. These data trades incorporate signs from the gut. Microscopic organisms in the gut can create concoction signals. These can follow up on the vagus nerve, shooting signals back to the mind. This might be one way that microscopic organisms in the gut can impact the state of mind. Invigorating the vagus straightforwardly has even been appeared to treat a few instances of serious despondency.

When is VNS used to treat epilepsy?

Synapses impart by sending an electrical flag in a precise example. In individuals with epilepsy, this example is, in some cases, upset due either to damage or the individual's hereditary make-up, causing synapses to discharge flag in an uncontrolled manner. This makes over-fervor, fairly like an electrical over-burden in the cerebrum, prompting seizures. Seizures can be delivered by electrical driving forces from all through the mind, called summed up seizures, or from a little region of the cerebrum, called incomplete seizures.

The vast majority with epilepsy can control their seizures with meds called hostile to convulsant or against seizure drugs.

About 20% of individuals with epilepsy don't react to hostile to seizure meds.

Sometimes, a medical procedure to expel the piece of the cerebrum causing the seizures might be utilized.

VNS might be a treatment choice for individuals whose seizures are not constrained by hostile to seizure meds and who are not viewed as a great possibility for a medical procedure; for instance, if their seizures are delivered all through the cerebrum (summed up).

How does VNS work?

It isn't known precisely how VNS functions. It is known, nonetheless, that the vagus nerve is a significant pathway to the cerebrum. It is imagined that by invigorating the vagus nerve, electrical vitality is released upward into a wide region of the mind, upsetting the irregular cerebrum action answerable for seizures. Another hypothesis proposes that invigorating the vagus nerve causes the arrival of uncommon mind synthetics that are diminishing seizure action.

What occurs during VNS? How is it performed?

While the patient is snoozing (general anesthesia), the triggering gadget (that is about the size of a silver dollar) is precisely put under the skin in the upper piece of the chest. An interfacing wire is run under the skin from the trigger to a terminal that is joined to the vagus nerve, which is open through a little entry point (cut) in the neck.

After it is embedded, the trigger is modified utilizing a PC to produce beats of power at ordinary interims, contingent upon the patient's resistance. For instance, the gadget might be modified to animate the nerve for 30 seconds at regular intervals. The settings on the gadget are movable, and the electrical flow is bitten by bit expanded as the patient's resistance increments. Reprogramming the trigger should be possible in the specialist's office. The patient likewise is given a hand-held magnet, which, when brought close to the trigger, can produce a quick flow of power to stop a seizure in advance or decrease the seriousness of the seizure.

VNS is an extra treatment, which implies it is utilized, notwithstanding another kind of treatment. Patients who experience VNS keep on taking their seizure meds. Now and again, be that as it may, it might be conceivable to diminish the dose of prescription.

IT'S CLICHE, BUT TAKE DEEP BREATHS

There's an association between breath and pulse, which is balanced by the vagus nerve. That's the reason customary yoga practice decreases by and large stress.

Yoga breathing and guided breathing activities, quiet your pulse, and lower your blood pressure. Breathing activities expanded vagal tone and viably oversaw prehypertension in a trial group.

In one examination, slow breathing activities improved autonomic capacities in sound members. Quick breathing didn't. That's since quick breathing makes your body believe you're running from predators. That sets off your body's alerts and enacts a pressure reaction.

In case you're terrified or going to blow a gasket, attempt box relaxing.

- Breathe in for a check of four.
- Hold for a check of four.
- Breathe out for a check of four.
- Sit tight for a check of four.
- Rehash until your hands are back on the controls.

A principal couple of times, follow your finger in a square example noticeable all around. It'll assist you with recollecting how to do it when you're fatigued.

The moderate development of your lungs sign to your heart to back off, which sends a sentiment of quiet all through your whole sensory system. Your vagus nerve associates the entirety of this flagging and discharges acetylcholine, a quieting substance you can give yourself a fix of whenever by doing unwinding methods.

Becoming accustomed to the virus conditions the vagus reaction, which eases back the initiation of the thoughtful sensory system. Standard virus impacts quantifiably decrease pressure markers. Cold introduction diminished indications of gloom and tension, potentially regulated by the vagus nerve.

Invigorating the vagal pathways animates digestion. When rodents' processing backed off because of uneasiness, cold introduction re-enacted the gastric nerves and got everything going once more. Everything occurred through vagal pathways.

KEEP YOUR GUT HAPPY

Have you ever known about the gut-mind hub? That alludes to the microorganisms in your stomach related framework speaking with your cerebrum.

Your microbiome is the biological system of agreeable microscopic organisms in your body and on your skin. Frequently, when somebody discusses the microbiome, they're discussing the organisms in your digestion tracts and colon.

As the study of the microbiome constructs, established researchers investigate an ever-increasing number of ways the microbiome influences your whole body. Research on the association between the microbiome and temperament is extending, and correspondence among gut and mind depends on — shock — the vagus nerve.

Concentrates on creature models and people bolster the possibility that a flourishing microbiome controls nervousness and improves your state of mind. A portion of the exploration analyzed this impact with and without a flawless vagus nerve, to check whether vagal pathways have anything to do with it.

Rodents who enhanced with specific strains of probiotics demonstrated abatements in nervousness and misery pointers, however not in creatures whose vagus nerves were cut before the experiment.

Analysts see the helpful impacts of probiotics on temperament in humans. Healthy ladies who ate matured nourishments for about a month indicated positive changes in mind movement, especially in the pieces of the cerebrum that control feeling and sensation. From the creature thinks about, and from what researchers think about the vagus nerve as of now, you can make strong speculation that the gut-mind correspondence here occurs through the vagus nerve.

The ideal approach to help your intestinal greenery is to get a far-reaching microbiome test like Viome. Viome is a test-at-home pack that you use to profile your microbiome effectively, and afterward, you get customized dietary suggestions to bring you once more into balance.

Discover YOUR SAFETY CUES

Vagus nerve master Dr. Stephen Porges set up Polyvagal Theory (more on that on a scene of Bulletproof Radio), which spreads out a choice procedure of sorts that decides if battle or-flight initiates. You are not aware of this procedure — everything occurs out of sight, and various parts of the vagus nerve initiate because of various circumstances.

At the point when you experience a terrifying improvement, the principal layer to traverse is the one that reacts to social correspondence — verbal language, non-verbal communication, vocal tone, and other nonverbal cues. If the boost is too solid to even think about reasoning through, your cerebrum actuates the battle or flight reaction. At the point when that falls flat, the crudest dread reaction is playing possum — feeling solidified.

At the point when you realize your dread is unreasonable, you can utilize security signals to stop alarm at the principal layer, and shield your cerebrum from getting to the battle or flight reaction. Here are a few things you can attempt.

Utilize SOOTHING VOICES

In his meeting on Bulletproof Radio, Stephen Porges clarifies one way this marvel is designed in kids. Youngsters are quantifiably quieted by prosodic (sing-songy) talking, otherwise called "motherese." Waldorf schools train educators to embrace this tone to keep up a quiet and upbeat homeroom. On the off chance that you've visited your local play area in the first part of the day, you've seen it in real life.

Changing your tone of discourse works for grown-ups, as well. Guided reflections, either face to face or recorded, embrace a moderate, musical tone of talking. Utilizing the voice as an unwinding sign urges your cerebrum into a casual state quicker than an ordinary conversational tone would.

TRAIN YOUR OWN SAFETY CUES

With a little practice, you can prepare your psyche to have a sense of security. Security signals shield your dread and uneasiness reactions from kicking in.

One approach to do this is to make your "sheltered spot" or "upbeat spot" while you're quiet. To do this, you envision you're at a spot where you're totally quiet and feeling and serene. Use as a lot of tactile data as you can – envision the sights, smells, sounds, and so on.

Practice this perception frequently. That way, when you start feeling frightful or furious, you can start the "protected spot" absent a lot of exertion. It's there when you need it.

Deal with YOUR MYELIN

Your vagus nerve is myelinated, which implies it's canvassed in a defensive covering of fat that protects it and enables the sign to go through productively. At the point when myelin on any nerve separates, the nerve doesn't fill in also. Peruse this post to study how to cherish your myelin.

Carefully IMPLANTED ELECTRICAL VAGUS NERVE STIMULATOR

The vagus nerve initiates the resistant framework when you're battling something. Doctors utilize this information for treatment by invigorating the vagus nerve with power and pharmaceuticals to treat incendiary disorders. Doctors carefully embed electric vagus nerve triggers in patients with serious epilepsy or gloom since it hoses the aggravation response.

YOU CAN TONE YOUR BABY'S VAGUS NERVE

A few variables play into the infant's vagal tone. Children who are brought into the world untimely or destined to moms who had melancholy and tension during pregnancy have a low vagal tone.

In the event that you were experiencing a few things during pregnancy, don't stress. You can help tone your infant's vagal pathways with ordinary holding practices and cherishing care.

Cold showers ought to most likely hold up until junior is mature enough to consent to it. During the child years, newborn child back rub and kangaroo care (holding infant skin-to-skin) help children's vagal tone develop. If your children are past the infant arrange, you can work with them on a portion of the adult approaches to condition the vagus nerve, such as breathing strategies and cold impacts in the shower.

A back rub, a yoga class, and a couple of moments of goosebumps in the shower are presumably justified, despite all the trouble thinking about that the advantages of vagal nerve conditioning reach out to each significant organ in your body and back. For more approaches to help your entire framework, head-to-toe, pop your data into the case underneath so you don't miss a thing.

The vagus nerve is one of 12 sets of cranial nerves that begin in mind and is a piece of the autonomic sensory system, which controls automatic body capacities. The nerve goes through the neck as it goes between the chest and mid-region, and the lower some portion of the cerebrum. It is associated with the engine works in the voice box, stomach, stomach, and heart and tangible capacities in the ears and tongue. It is associated with both engine and tangible capacities in the sinuses and throat.

Vagus nerve incitement (VNS) sends normal, gentle beats of electrical vitality to the mind by means of the vagus nerve through a gadget that is like a pacemaker. There is no physical contribution of the cerebrum in this medical procedure and patients can't by and large feel the beats. It is imperative to remember that VNS is a treatment choice constrained to choose people with epilepsy or treatment-safe gloom.

This strategy, performed by a neurosurgeon, normally takes around 45-an hour and a half with the patient most ordinarily under general anesthesia. It is generally performed on an outpatient premise. Likewise, with all medical procedures, there is little danger of contamination. Other careful dangers of VNS incorporate aggravation or torment at the entry point site, harm to close by nerves, and nerve tightening.

The method requires two little entry points. The first is made on the upper left half of the chest, where the beat generator is embedded. A subsequent entry point is made on a level plane on the left half of the lower neck, along a wrinkle of skin. This is the place the slight, adaptable wires that associate the beat generator to the vagus nerve are embedded.

The vagus nerve gives a fast line of data to the mind from the gut, where fights with microorganisms and infections are persistently seething. Information on the vagus' job was a puzzle until as of late, yet we presently realize that you can find out about your body from your vagus.

The longest nerve legitimately from the mind, the vagus sends messages to and gets messages from your gut and each other organ in your body. Since 85 percent of this colossal nerve conveys data back to the cerebrum, it's the fundamental instrument by which your mind reviews your body. The staying 15 percent takes data from your mind to your body.

One of the key procedures in this messaging framework includes Toll-like receptors, which animate an invulnerable reaction once trespassers have ruptured a zone like the skin or gut. The microbes are colonizing our gut work to square new microscopic organisms from moving into the area.

The toll receptors can recognize successfully between pathogen cells and host cells, and they fill in as a kind of smoke caution for your body by putting your safe framework on ready when outside cells have attacked, with the goal that the safe group can deal with them before any harm happens. Be that as it may, this early cautioning framework is a crude guard and comes up short on the modernity of a portion of the other insusceptible cells.

How does the vagus nerve influence wellbeing?

While we realize the vagus nerve has numerous capacities, we're not in every case totally sure how it functions. What we do know: It's a key player in the parasympathetic sensory system. The more we invigorate the vagus nerve (by profound breathing, for instance), the more we upgrade the quieting impacts of the parasympathetic (or "rest and overview") sensory system and counter the animating impacts of the thoughtful (or "battle or flight") sensory system.

The vagus nerve is additionally a scaffold by which the enteric sensory system (or ENS, which oversees the capacity of the GI tract) speaks with the focal sensory system (CNS). Together, the ENS and CNS work to control the development of the GI tract, its emissions, invulnerable capacity for microbes, and bloodstream.

Which is all to state, how well the vagus nerve is working—and hence, how well the gut and the mind are conveying—can affect everything from uneasiness levels to pulse to assimilation to weight increase, and substantially more.

What causes your vagus nerve to fail to meet expectations.

Poor vagal tone or working can have huge wellbeing suggestions. Interruption of vagus nerve capacity can be brought about by unnecessary pressure, sickness, certain prescriptions, aggravation, and diseases, in addition to other things—and when upset, the body has a general progressively troublesome time unwinding and taking care of its essential capacities including resting, breathing, processing, and development of squanders by means of the GI tract, lungs, and skin.

In addition to other things, this poor vagal working can prompt stagnation and bacterial abundance in the GI tract, and, thusly, these "terrible" gut microorganisms may impact the action of the nerve center pituitary-adrenal (HPA) pivot by means of the vagus nerve, which can influence significant neuronal cell action in mind and lead to aggravation and neurodegeneration, which demonstrates how it's everything associated.

Yet, that is not all. Here are some different issues related to the low vagal tone, or a failure to meet expectations vagus nerve:

- Sickness
- Regurgitating
- Looseness of the bowels
- Clogging

- Gastroparesis
- Reflux
- Uneasiness and sadness
- Weight gain
- Stomach torment
- Joint and muscle torment
- Cerebral pains
- Psychosis
- Memory misfortune
- Temperature dysregulation
- Discombobulation
- Weariness
- A sleeping disorder

The most effective method to improve gut-mind correspondence by means of the vagus nerve and lift in general wellbeing.

Luckily, there are a few things we can do without anyone else to advance the correspondence between the cerebrum and the gut by method for the vagus nerve. The means delineated beneath can help manage vagal tone, diminish aggravation (which can smother vagus nerve work), and guarantee in general solid parasympathetic and thoughtful equalization. This, thusly, can assist you with recouping all the more rapidly after times of pressure, improve assimilation, and lead to a large group of other full-body benefits.

1. Attempt profound breathing or reflection

Profound breathing is one of the most basic yet compelling approaches to animate the vagus nerve. When you breath out is even a couple of checks longer than you breathe in, the vagus nerve sends a sign to your mind to turn up your parasympathetic sensory system. Attempt this activity: Breath for two excludes in, and four checks out, with one tally stop at the highest point of the breath in and a one tally delay at the base of the breath out. Various investigations likewise bolster the intensity of reflection to improve torment, rest, craving, nervousness, and gastrointestinal capacity through an immediate impact on vagal tone.

2. Head to a yoga class.

Research shows that taking part in customary moderate exercise, for example, yoga increments gastric motility—the constrictions of the smooth gastric muscle basic for the development of nourishment through the stomach related tract—and that it does this by method for invigorating the vagus nerve.

Consider finishing your shower with a one-minute impact of cold water, and don't be reluctant to set out outside toward a walk when it's crisp. Studies show that intense cold introduction initiates the vagus nerve, just as different neurons on the vagus nerve pathway, causing a move toward parasympathetic sensory system action.

3. Clean up.

Consider finishing your shower with a one-minute impact of cold water, and don't be reluctant to set out outside toward a walk when it's nippy. Studies show that intense cold presentation initiates the vagus nerve, just as different neurons on the vagus nerve pathway, causing a move toward parasympathetic sensory system action.

4. Eat nourishments wealthy in tryptophan.

Dietary tryptophan is utilized in the gut and may support the astrocytes—cells in the cerebrum and spinal string—control irritation, which may improve correspondence from the gut to the mind through the vagal envoy pathway. These nourishments incorporate spinach, seeds, nuts, bananas, and poultry.

5. Keep up a sound weight.

Stoutness and gut aggravation can upset the vagal movement and adversely influence the association between the mind and the GI tract. So in case, you're overweight, your most logical option is to embrace economical practices that will prompt long haul weight reduction. My recommendation: Move your body day by day and spotlight on expending an eating routine high in an assortment of vegetables and organic products, alongside nuts, seeds, and vegetables, for example, the Mediterranean eating routine.

6. Ensure you crap day by day.

Expend a lot of fiber-rich nourishments day by day (go for 25 or more grams), and keep up routine rest and exercise examples to enable your body to dispense with on a day by day musicality. Solid disposal guarantees less stagnation of incendiary nourishment buildups in the colon and a less neighborly condition for undesirable living beings that can impede correspondence between the mind and gut.

7. Nix sugar from your eating regimen.

Unnecessary sugar causes constant irritation as well as weakens cell criticism circles and other flagging pathways, and aggravation of the GI tract mucosal covering enables pathogens to propagate fiery sign to the cerebrum additionally.

8. Pop a probiotic.

Notwithstanding cutting your admission of sugar to cultivate a sound gut and keep up ideal gut-cerebrum flagging, consider including matured nourishments or a probiotic to your eating routine.

Research shows that gut microorganisms can really actuate the vagus nerve. In one examination, mice that were given the probiotic Lactobacillus rhamnosus experienced expanded GABA creation and a decrease in pressure, misery, and nervousness. Be that as it may, this gainful impact didn't happen among mice whose vagus nerve had been evacuated.

9. In the event that you eat heaps of creature protein, downsize.

Red meat and eggs contain choline, which can be beneficial for you, yet when devoured in overabundance is changed over to trimethylamine N-oxide (TMAO), an aggravate that has been related with irritation and cardiovascular issues. Diminished utilization of these nourishments may diminish aggravation and permit the vagus nerve to all the more likely control parasympathetic and thoughtful vitals, for example, circulatory strain and pulse.

10. Think about discontinuous fasting.

A few investigations propose that fasting and dietary confinement can enact the vagus nerve. What's more, given fasting's host of different advantages—from improved intellectual capacity to weight reduction to decreased irritation—it might merit an attempt. The best part: Your fasting window shouldn't be that long to receive some incredible rewards.

11. Belt out your preferred tune.

Research shows that singing has a naturally mitigating impact, which has an inseparable tie to the vagus nerve. So proceed, chime into the radio when you're in the vehicle—or even better, when you're scrubbing down!

These are only a couple of things you can do to improve mind work, gut work, and everything in the middle. Now and again, complex pathways can react to straightforward intercessions.

Barriers to Vagus Nerve while functioning

Despite the fact that the gastrointestinal (GI) tract contains inborn neural plexuses that permit a critical level of autonomous power over GI works, the focal sensory system gives outward neural information sources that adjust, direct, and incorporate these capacities. Specifically, the vagus nerve (VN) gives the parasympathetic innervation to the GI tract, co-ordinates the mind-boggling connections among focal and fringe neural control systems.

Intestinal penetrability annoyance is a marvel that is by and large progressively perceived as a contributing variable to a huge number of sicknesses - including incendiary inside ailment (IBD) and bad-tempered entrail disorder (IBS). There are right now restricted successful treatment techniques known to improve this intestinal porousness annoyance, and the utilization of vagal nerve incitement would introduce itself as an economical, non-intrusive, and nonpharmacological strategy for switching this brokenness. Vagal nerve incitement adequacy in turning around pressure-related intestinal boundary brokenness is accessible from the verification of idea creature models.

Chapter Five: Relations between vagus nerves and parasympathetic system

Step by step instructions to Hack Your Nervous System

The vagus nerve is the most significant nerve you presumably didn't have any acquaintance with you had.

In contrast to different Vegas, what occurs in this vagus doesn't remain there. The vagus nerve is a long wandering heap of the engine and tactile strands that connections the cerebrum stem to the heart, lungs, and gut. It likewise fans out to contact and connect with the liver, spleen, gallbladder, ureter, female richness organs, neck, ears, tongue, and kidneys. It controls up our automatic operational hub—the parasympathetic sensory system—and controls oblivious body capacities, just as everything from keeping our pulse steady and nourishment processing to breathing and perspiring. It likewise directs pulse and blood glucose balance, advances general kidney work, helps discharge bile and testosterone, invigorates the emission of salivation, helps with controlling taste and discharging tears, and assumes a significant job in ripeness issues and climaxes in ladies.

Dr. Justin Hoffman, a Santa Rosa, California, authorized naturopathic medicinal doctor, says:

Without the vagus nerve, key capacities that keep us alive would not be kept up.

Broadly perceived games nutritionist, quality, and molding mentor Brandon Mentore explains:

The vagus nerve is incredibly basic to your general wellbeing and is personally connected to different organs and frameworks of the body. The vagus nerve has strands that innervate for all intents and purposes the entirety of our inside organs. The administration and handling of feelings happen through the vagal nerve between the heart, mind, and gut, which is the reason we have a solid gut response to serious mental and passionate states.

Passionate processing Emotional handling happens by means of the vagal nerve between the heart, mind, and gut.

Vagus nerve brokenness can bring about an entire host of issues, including heftiness, bradycardia (unusually moderate heartbeat), trouble gulping, gastrointestinal sicknesses, blacking out, disposition issue, B12 lack, constant irritation, disabled hack, and seizures.

In the interim, the vagus nerve incitement has been appeared to improve conditions, for example,

- Tension issue
- Coronary illness
- Tinnitus
- Stoutness
- Liquor fixation
- Headaches
- Alzheimer's
- Cracked gut

- Ill will dissemination
- State of mind issue
- Malignancy
- A Closer Look At This Super Nerve

The vagus nerve is the longest of our 12 cranial nerves. Just the spinal section is a bigger nerve framework. Around 80 percent of its nerve strands—or four of its five 'paths'— drive data from the body to the mind. Its fifth path runs the other way, moving sign from the cerebrum all through the body. Moored in the mind stem, the vagus goes through the neck and into the chest, parting into the left vagus and the correct vagus. Every one of these streets is made out of countless nerve filaments that branch into the heart, lungs, stomach, pancreas, and almost every other organ in the mid-region. The vagus nerve utilizes the synapse acetylcholine, which animates muscle compressions in the parasympathetic sensory system. A synapse is a sort of compound delivery person discharged toward the finish of a nerve fiber, that takes into consideration sign to be moved along from point to point, which invigorates different organs. For instance, if our mind couldn't speak with our stomach through the arrival of acetylcholine from the vagus nerve, at that point, we would quit relaxing.

The longest cranial nerve vagus nerve is the longest of our 12 cranial nerves.

A few substances, for example, botox and the overwhelming metal mercury, can meddle with acetylcholine creation. Botox has been known to close down the vagus nerve, which causes demise. Mercury hinders the activity of acetylcholine. At the point when mercury appends to the thiol protein in the heart muscle receptors, the heart muscle can't get the vagus nerve electrical drive for compression. Cardiovascular issues ordinarily pursue. Mercury utilized in fillings just crawls from the mind just as the 3,000 tons of mercury put into the air can meddle with acetylcholine creation. Mercury-loaded antibodies may likewise assume a job in vagus nerve-related mental imbalance in youngsters.

Hoffman says:

Hypothetically, anything that improves the nearness and capacity of acetylcholine will likewise manage the strength of our vagus nerve.

He prescribes common nootropics huperzine and galantamine for improving the affectability of acetylcholine receptors.

Vagus nerve harm can likewise be brought about by diabetes, liquor abuse, upper respiratory viral contaminations, or having some portion of the nerve cut off incidentally during an activity. Stress can kindle the nerve, alongside weakness and uneasiness. In any event, something as straightforward as a terrible stance can adversely affect the vagus nerve.

Copious proof connections thoughtful sensory system initiation to results of patients with a cardiovascular breakdown (HF). Conversely, parasympathetic actuation has complex cardiovascular impacts that are just starting to be perceived. Specifically, the pathophysiological jobs of ordinary and cluttered parasympathetic innervation in patients with HF are not comprehended as comprehensively.

In the present, we audit cardiovascular reactions to parasympathetic enactment, address the adjusting factors that can influence parasympathetic capacity, talk about the job of the vagus nerve in ventricular brokenness, and think about how actuation of the parasympathetic sensory system may have significant remedial ramifications for patients with congestive HF.

Structure of the Parasympathetic Limb of the Autonomic Nervous System

The parasympathetic sensory system starts from average medullary locales (core questionable, core tractus solitarius, and dorsal engine core) and is tweaked by the nerve center. Vagal efferents stretch out from the medulla to postganglionic nerves that innervate the atria by means of ganglia situated in heart fat cushions with neurotransmission that is tweaked by means of nicotinic receptors. Postganglionic parasympathetic and thoughtful cholinergic nerves at that point influence cardiovascular muscarinic receptors.

Vagus nerve afferent enactment, beginning incidentally, can balance efferent thoughtful and parasympathetic capacity midway and at the degree of the baroreceptor. Efferent vagus nerve actuation can have tonic and basal impacts that hinder thoughtful initiation and arrival of norepinephrine at the presynaptic level. Acetylcholine discharge from parasympathetic nerve terminals will initiate ganglionic nicotinic receptors that thus actuate muscarinic receptors at the cell level. Cardiovascular impacts incorporate pulse decrease by restraint of the thoughtful sensory system and by direct hyperpolarization of sinus nodal cells. Parasympathetic actuation can influence atrioventricular nodal conduction interceded prevalently through the left vagus nerve. Moreover, muscarinic receptors on vein dividers can cause vasorelaxation through nitric oxide (NO)– tweaked pathway, however, can likewise cause vasoconstriction by straightforwardly initiating smooth muscle.6–8 Therefore, in spite of the fact that the thoughtful sensory system effects affect cardiovascular physiology in an all-or-none kind of reaction, the parasympathetic sensory system can have a particular balance at different levels.

Parasympathetic/Sympathetic Interactions

The thoughtful and parasympathetic sensory systems are not "alternate extremes"; rather, the connections are complex.9 A powerful communication happens between them; these cooperations are adjusted halfway by optional dispatchers (cAMP and cGMP). The parasympathetic sensory system can hinder thoughtful nerve traffic presynaptically. In like manner, thoughtful enactment can restrain parasympathetic actuation presynaptically.

Vagal "tone" (tonic parasympathetic initiation) prevails over thoughtful tone very still. Under ordinary physiological conditions, unexpected parasympathetic incitement will repress thoughtful tonic actuation and its belongings very still and during exercise. This reaction is known as "highlighted antagonism."10–12 In a static13 or dynamic14 state, a raised thoughtful tone is superseded by extreme vagus nerve release.

In HF, perceptions in ventricular myocardium show at the degree of heart myocyte work give experiences into the relationship of thoughtful and parasympathetic capacity. The impact of intracoronary acetylcholine to restrain a β-adrenergic–invigorated increment in the primary subsidiary of left ventricular weight after some time is safeguarded, proposing that the post-receptor pathway is unblemished. Be that as it may, these equivalent investigations show a decrease in tonic parasympathetic actuation in HF on the grounds that intracoronary atropine expanded the reaction of the principal subsidiary of left ventricular weight after some time to dobutamine in typical patients (demonstrating nearness of huge parasympathetic tone) however not in HF (recommending less parasympathetic tone in the heart).

β-Adrenergic incitement causes apoptosis of heart myocytes. This impact, intervened by protein kinase An and requiring calcium section through voltage-subordinate calcium channels, may add to the movement of myocardial disappointment. Muscarinic receptor incitement contradicts this activity by a G(i)- interceded flagging pathway that restricts activities of adenylyl cyclase. Carbachol, a muscarinic agonist, can avoid β-adrenergic receptor–invigorated apoptosis, and along these lines may demonstrate that muscarinic actuation can improve results in HF by this mechanism.

Muscarinic Receptors

Muscarinic receptors live in both the atria and ventricles however have a more noteworthy thickness in the former.6 They happen more in the endocardium than in the epicardium. Muscarinic receptors exist on T tubules in cardiomyocytes, coronary supply routes (counting little vessels), and endothelial cell layers of vessels. Muscarinic receptors are rich in sinoatrial and atrioventricular nodal cells.

The known impacts of the parasympathetic sensory system on cardiovascular capacity, pulse, and atrioventricular nodal conduction seem adjusted for the most part by means of M2 receptors. M3 and M4 receptors might be colocalized on different cardiovascular structures, yet their job in tweaking quantifiable physiological reactions in people stays dubious. The distinctive muscarinic receptor subtypes can have various impacts. The M2 receptor will particularly slow the pulse (interceded to a limited extent by G-protein deep down correcting potassium [GIRK] channels), abbreviate atrial activity possibilities, increment smooth muscle constriction, hinder the amusing current, initiate the G-protein–gated atrial potassium channel (IKACh), and lessening contractility straightforwardly. The M3 and M4 receptors are upregulated in congestive HF; the previous can enact the potassium channel IKM3, and the last will actuate GIRK1 and IKACh.

Antibodies to the M2 receptor have been recognized in patients with widened cardiomyopathy and may impact the improvement of atrial fibrillation.5,21–25 In a creature model, autoantibodies have been related to redesigning in HF, yet it isn't sure how the two are related.26 M2 receptor power likewise was seen to move to M3 and M4 receptors. Cardiovascular M3 receptors may influence pulse and heart repolarization, balance inotropic impacts, ensure against ischemic damage, control cell-cell correspondence, and have antiarrhythmic and proarrhythmic effects.27 A potential job for the M3 receptor in starting and keeping up atrial fibrillation in HF has been proposed.28 M3 receptor enactment may opposite affect pulse contrasted and M2 receptor initiation. The job of M4 receptors remains unclear,29, yet they seem to tweak diverse repolarization flows.

Nicotinic Receptors

Nicotinic receptors live on the postganglionic parasympathetic neuron and hence can influence vagus nerve action. Nicotinic receptors don't straightforwardly invigorate or legitimately influence organs, yet they are liable for ganglionic transmission and at last, are answerable for end-organ parasympathetic initiation. Diminished synaptic transmission in parasympathetic ganglia may add to irregular parasympathetic capacity in HF. To a limited extent, weakened parasympathetic control in HF is situated inside the fringe efferent appendage inside the parasympathetic ganglion in a canine HF model.

Nicotinic receptors intervene in synaptic ganglionic transmission and upregulate in light of constant presentation to an agonist. Rehashed presentation of ganglionic neurons to a nicotinic agonist to counteract the loss of parasympathetic control in HF has been tried. Notwithstanding diminished ganglionic work prompting decreased parasympathetic control in HF, rehashed presentation to a nicotinic agonist during HF improvement brought about saved, even supernormal, impacts of parasympathetic stimulation.

Sorts of Vagus Nerve Fibers

A great part of the comprehension of the histology of the fiber type in the cervical vagus nerve is gotten from creatures (canine, cat, and other mammals). The vagus nerve tends to be indifferent sorts. Although contrasts can be found in the appropriation of the fascicles by species in the cervical vagus, the quantitative relations between the different kinds and elements of filaments are similar.4 Afferent strands prevail and incorporate gradually leading unmyelinated C strands and little width A-delta strands that underlie the vibe of alluded neck and jaw torment experienced in angina pectoris. The C filaments in efferent fascicles add to tonic cardio-hindrance and are interceded by muscarinic receptors. Efferent fascicles additionally contain huge myelinated A-beta filaments that have a place with the laryngeal pack and cardio-inhibitory A-delta strands that energize postganglionic neurons in the cardiovascular fat cushions by means of nicotinic receptors. Hypothetically, at any rate, particular incitement is expected to impact cardio-restraint without producing different impacts or inspiring pain.

Focal Influences on Parasympathetic Innervation

Parasympathetic innervation might be adjusted by various midway intervened instruments. Focal γ-aminobutyric corrosive (GABA) instruments may advance vagus nerve withdrawal. Specifically, apparently, GABA represses vagus nerve outflow40 interceded through the GABAB receptor. Centrally acting narcotics (enkephalins) interfere with vagus nerve–prompted bradycardia through a muscarinic impact. Mu-narcotic receptors and narcotic-like receptors (ORL-1) inside the core uncertain propose that narcotics balance synaptic transmission to cardiovascular vagal neurons. A mu-particular endogenous agonist, D-Ala2, N-Me-Phe4, Gly5-of-enkephalin (DAMGO), and nociceptin decline glycinergic contributions to vagal neurons in the core equivocal, proposing focal tweak of parasympathetic activation. Decreases in glycinergic transmission increment parasympathetic movement and might be a component by which narcotics prompt bradycardia as well as impact atrial fibrillation. Serotonin, neuropeptides, and even cannabinoids can adjust parasympathetic capacity centrally.

Pulse Control

As noted, pulse control by the parasympathetic sensory system is generally intricate. Enactment from the focal sensory system of vagal preganglionic nerves can, by means of nicotinic receptors, initiate the postganglionic vagal nerve. The ensuing arrival of acetylcholine invigorates the muscarinic receptors, which, thusly, actuate NO synthase (NOS) through guanylate cyclase to repress the L-type calcium channel. The M2 receptor can in a roundabout way, enact IKACh to slow the sinus rate. Furthermore, M2 receptors on the presynaptic thoughtful nerve terminal will hinder norepinephrine release.

Pulse and Outcomes

Resting pulse in an ordinary heart, for the most part, is administered by a parasympathetic system. Epidemiological information demonstrates that the resting pulse, a proportion of vagus nerve work, predicts mortality. The higher the vagus nerve action is, the slower the pulse is, the more noteworthy the expansion in the parasympathetic segment of pulse inconstancy is, and the better the result is. In HF, the pulse is less directed by parasympathetic initiation. A synopsis of information on the resting pulse and cardiovascular illness shows a strong connection between expanded pulse and antagonistic outcomes.

Assessment of Parasympathetic Activation

Parasympathetic capacity is hard to gauge legitimately. Parasympathetic impacts can be estimated roughly by reactions to vagus nerve incitement (Valsalva or comparable moves) and barricade (atropine or antimuscarinic, M2 receptor blocker) or physiological perceptions, for example, diminished pulse or respiratory sinus arrhythmia. Progressively refined estimations are correspondingly roundabout and noninvasive, for example, assessment of pulse changeability, pulse recuperation from exercise, and ghastly turbulence.

A few lines of proof recommend that pulse changeability is a marker, yet vague, of autonomic tone and that pulse disturbance, might be a marker of baroreceptor sensitivity. The high-recurrence segments of pulse inconstancy are related to vagus nerve/parasympathetic impact, while the low-recurrence parts are because of thoughtful and parasympathetic enactment. Of note, contrasts exist between the proportions of low-recurrence to high-recurrence segments, contingent upon the reason for HF. Baroreflex affectability, which reflects partially parasympathetic innervation, likewise is hard to quantify straightforwardly. It might reflect focal vagal yield and incorporate contribution from the carotid sinus, aortic and atrial receptors, and left ventricular (LV) mechanoreceptors.

Change of Parasympathetic Control in HF

Parasympathetic enactment and its physiological impacts are lessened in HF. The information demonstrates that adjustments in vagus nerve control of pulse become evident at an early formative phase of LV brokenness, which may give significant prognostic data in patients in danger for creating dynamic myocardial dysfunction.

In HF, the vagal ganglionic transmission is diminished, muscarinic receptor thickness and synthesis are adjusted, and acetylcholinesterase movement is diminished. In test HF, a muscarinic barricade has an increasingly humble impact on pulse contrasted and controls. Muscarinic receptor bar increments heart norepinephrine overflow when HF is absent; however, a blunting of parasympathetic effect on thoughtful movement is available in HF.

Alternately, LV muscarinic incitement has an autonomous negative lusitropic impact and alienates β-adrenergic stimulation. Reduced vagus nerve control might be because of changes in the presynaptic (ganglionic) function. Muscarinic receptor enactment by bethanechol (direct muscarinic incitement) and in a roundabout way by neostigmine (an acetylcholinesterase inhibitor) inspired overstated pulse responses. Abnormal baroreflex control of pulse in patients with HF is well recognized. Evidence additionally exists for hindrance of vagally intervened baroreflex bradycardia on the grounds that vagal neurons with ordinary systolic weight levels have a lower resting release rate.

Pulse changes in light of preganglionic and postganglionic parasympathetic sinus hub incitement in hounds with HF show that diminished vagus nerve control in HF is because of strange presynaptic components, perhaps including anomalous capacity at the degree of the ganglion.30 Lack of weakening of thoughtful incitement by the parasympathetic sensory system can be watched, which is brought about by variations from the norm in cardiopulmonary baroreceptors, focal abnormalities, changes in the communications between the thoughtful and parasympathetic appendages, adjustments at the nicotinic ganglionic level, or changes in the muscarinic receptors. In tissue tests from explanted bombed human hearts, the absence of weakening and ceaseless β-adrenergic incitement prompts an expanded articulation of Giα-mRNA and G(i) protein and to an upgraded power of the negative inotropic impact of muscarinic agonists, recommending an input component changing parasympathetic influences.

Vagus nerve afferent enactment may add to the actuation of the neurohumoral frameworks. Specifically, vagal afferents actuated during HF may add to raised degrees of vasopressin and sympathoexcitation.

Chapter Six: How to treat symptoms naturally

Vagus nerve incitement includes the utilization of a gadget to animate the vagus nerve with electrical motivations. An implantable vagus nerve trigger is, as of now, FDA-endorsed to treat epilepsy and sadness. There's one vagus nerve on each side of your body, running from your brainstem through your neck to your chest and stomach area.

In ordinary vagus nerve incitement, a gadget is carefully embedded under the skin on your chest, and a wire is strung under your skin, interfacing the gadget to one side vagus nerve. At the point when initiated, the gadget sends an electrical flag along the left vagus nerve to your brainstem, which at that point, sends a sign to specific regions in your mind. The correct vagus nerve isn't utilized in light of the fact that it's bound to convey strands that supply nerves to the heart.

New, noninvasive vagus nerve incitement gadgets, which don't require careful implantation, have been affirmed in Europe to treat epilepsy, sadness, and torment. A noninvasive gadget that animates the vagus nerve was as of late endorsed by the Food and Drug Administration for the treatment of group migraines in the United States.

Around 33% of individuals with epilepsy don't completely react to hostile to seizure drugs. Vagus nerve incitement might be a choice to diminish the recurrence of seizures in individuals who haven't accomplished control with meds.

Vagus nerve incitement may likewise be useful for individuals who haven't reacted to escalated melancholy medicines, for example, energizer prescriptions, mental guiding (psychotherapy), and electroconvulsive treatment (ECT).

The Food and Drug Administration (FDA) has endorsed vagus nerve incitement for individuals who:

- Have central (incomplete) epilepsy

- Have seizures that aren't well-controlled with meds

The FDA has likewise endorsed vagus nerve incitement for the treatment of sorrow in grown-ups who:

Have ceaseless, difficult-to-treat melancholy (treatment-safe despondency)

Haven't improved in the wake of attempting at least four prescriptions or electroconvulsive treatment (ECT), or both

Proceed with standard sorrow medicines alongside vagus nerve incitement

Moreover, specialists are examining vagus nerve incitement as a potential treatment for an assortment of conditions, including cerebral pains, rheumatoid joint inflammation, provocative entrail infection, bipolar issue, heftiness, and Alzheimer's ailment.

Dangers

For a great many people, vagus nerve incitement is protected. In any case, it has a few dangers, both from the medical procedure to embed the gadget and from the mind incitement.

Medical procedure dangers

Careful complexities with embedded vagus nerve incitement are uncommon and are like the threats of having different kinds of medical procedures. They include:

Torment where the (cut) is made to embed the gadget

Disease

Trouble gulping

Vocal rope loss of motion, which is normally transitory, yet can be lasting

Reactions after a medical procedure

A portion of the reactions and medical issues related to embedded vagus nerve incitement can include:

- Voice changes
- Raspiness
- Throat torment
- Hack
- Cerebral pains
- Brevity of breath
- Trouble gulping
- Shivering or prickling of the skin
- A sleeping disorder
- Declining of rest apnea

For the vast majority, reactions are passable. They may reduce after some time, yet some symptoms may stay irksome for whatever length of time that you utilize embedded vagus nerve incitement.

Changing the electrical driving forces can help limit these impacts. In the event that symptoms are unfortunate, the gadget can be closed off briefly or for all time.

How you plan

It's imperative to deliberately consider the upsides and downsides of embedded vagus nerve incitement before choosing to have the technique. Ensure you realize what the entirety of your other treatment decisions are and that you and your primary care physician both feel that embedded vagus nerve incitement is the best choice for you. Ask your primary care physician precisely what you ought to expect during a medical procedure and after they beat generator is set up.

Nourishment and drugs

You may need to quit taking certain drugs early, and your PCP may ask you not to eat the night prior to the system.

What you can anticipate

Prior to the methodology

Prior to a medical procedure, your PCP will do a physical assessment. You may require blood tests or different tests to ensure you don't have any wellbeing worries that may be an issue. Your primary care physician may have you start taking anti-microbials before medical procedures to avoid disease.

During the technique

Medical procedure to embed the vagus nerve incitement gadget should be possible on an outpatient premise. However, a few specialists suggest remaining medium-term.

The medical procedure, for the most part, takes an hour to 90 minutes. You may stay conscious yet have drugs to numb the medical procedure territory (nearby anesthesia), or you might be oblivious during the medical procedure (general anesthesia).

The medical procedure itself doesn't include your mind. Two cuts are made, one on your chest or in the armpit (axillary) district, and the other on the left half of the neck.

The beat generator is embedded in the upper left half of your chest. The gadget is intended to be a perpetual embed. However, it tends to be expelled if important.

The beat generator is about the size of a stopwatch and runs on battery control. A lead wire is associated with the heartbeat generator. The lead wire is guided under your skin from your chest up to your neck, where it's appended to one side vagus nerve during that time entry point.

After the methodology

The beat generator is turned on during a visit to your primary care physician's office half a month after a medical procedure. At that point, it very well may be customized to convey electrical motivations to the vagus nerve at different terms, frequencies, and flows. Vagus nerve incitement, for the most part, begins at a low level and is slowly expanded, contingent upon your indications and reactions.

Incitement is customized to turn on and off in explicit cycles —, for example, 30 seconds on, five minutes off. You may make them shiver sensations or slight genuine annoyance and transitory dryness when the nerve incitement is on.

The trigger doesn't recognize seizure action or melancholy side effects. At the point when it's turned on, the trigger turns on and off at the interims chose by your PCP. You can utilize a hand-held magnet to start incitement at an alternate time, for instance, in the event that you sense a looming seizure.

The magnet can likewise be utilized to incidentally kill the vagus nerve incitement, which might be essential when you do certain exercises, for example, open talking, singing, or working out, or when you're eating in the event that you have gulping issues.

You'll have to visit your primary care physician occasionally to ensure that the beat generator is working accurately and that it hasn't moved out of position. Check with your primary care physician before having any restorative tests, for example, attractive reverberation imaging (MRI), which may meddle with your gadget.

Results

Embedded vagus nerve incitement isn't a solution for epilepsy. A great many people with epilepsy won't quit having seizures or taking epilepsy medicine inside and out after the methodology. However, many will have fewer seizures, up to 20 to 50 percent less. Seizure force may diminish too.

It can take months or even a year or longer of incitement before you see any critical decrease in seizures. Vagus nerve incitement may likewise abbreviate the recuperation time after a seizure. Individuals who've had vagus nerve incitement to treat epilepsy may likewise encounter upgrades in disposition and personal satisfaction.

Research is as yet blended on the advantages of embedded vagus nerve incitement for the treatment of discouragement. A few investigations recommend the advantages of vagus nerve incitement for discouragement gather after some time, and it might take at any rate a while of treatment before you see any enhancements in your downturn side effects. Embedded vagus nerve incitement doesn't work for everyone, and it isn't proposed to supplant conventional medicines.

Fiery reactions assume a focal job in the advancement and determination of numerous ailments and can prompt incapacitating ceaseless torment. As a rule, aggravation is your body's reaction to push. In this way, decreasing "battle or-flight" reactions in the sensory system and bringing down organic markers for stress can likewise diminish irritation.

Ordinarily, specialists endorse prescriptions to battle irritation. Nonetheless, there's developing proof that another method to battle irritation is by connecting with the vagus nerve and improving "vagal tone." This can be accomplished through every day propensities, for example, yoga and contemplation—or in progressively outrageous instances of aggravation, for example, rheumatoid joint inflammation (RA)— by utilizing an embedded gadget for vagus nerve incitement (VNS).

The vagus nerve is known as the "meandering nerve" since it has different branches that veer from two thick stems established in the cerebellum and brainstem that meander to the least viscera of your belly contacting your heart and most significant organs en route. Vagus signifies "meandering" in Latin. The words drifter, ambiguous, and transient are altogether gotten from a similar Latin root.

In 1921, a German physiologist named Otto Loewi found that animating the vagus nerve caused a decrease in pulse by setting off the arrival of a substance he instituted Vagusstoff (German for "Vagus Substance"). The "vagus substance" was later distinguished as acetylcholine and turned into the primary synapse at any point recognized by researchers.

Vagusstoff (acetylcholine) resembles a sedative that you can self-direct essentially by taking a couple of full breaths with long breathes out. Deliberately taking advantage of the intensity of your vagus nerve can make a condition of internal quiet while subduing your irritation reflex.

The vagus nerve is the prime segment of the parasympathetic sensory system, which directs the "rest-and-digest" or "tend-and-get to know" reactions. On the other side, to look after homeostasis, the thoughtful sensory system drives the "battle or flight" reaction.

Sound vagal tone is shown by a slight increment of the pulse when you breathe in, and a reduction of the pulse when you breathe out. Profound diaphragmatic breathing—with a long, slow breathe out—is vital to invigorating the vagus nerve and easing back pulse and circulatory strain, particularly in the midst of execution nervousness.

A higher vagal tone record is connected to physical and mental prosperity. Alternately, a low vagal tone list is related to aggravation, sadness, negative states of mind, forlornness, coronary failures, and stroke.

A recent report, "How Positive Emotions Build Physical Health: Perceived Positive Social

Connections Account for the Upward Spiral Between Positive Emotions and Vagal Tone," was distributed in Psychological Science. For this examination, Barbara Fredrickson and Bethany Kok of the University of North Carolina at Chapel Hill focused on the vagus nerve and found that a high vagal tone record was a piece of a criticism circle between positive feelings, physical wellbeing, and positive social associations.

Their examination proposes that positive feelings, powerful social associations, and physical wellbeing impact each other in a self-supporting upward winding dynamic and input circle that researchers are simply starting to comprehend.

For this examination, Frederickson and Kok utilized a Loving-Kindness Meditation (LKM) method to assist members with getting better at self-producing positive feelings. In any case, they additionally found that essentially considering positive social associations and attempting to improve affectionate human bonds likewise caused enhancements in vagal tone.

In 2014, I composed a Psychology Today blog entry, "How Does the Vagus Nerve Convey Gut Instincts to the Brain?" in view of discoveries by specialists in Switzerland who recognized how the vagus nerve passes on "premonitions" of nervousness and dread to the mind. Clinical and trial contemplates showing that pressure and melancholy are related with the up-guideline of the resistant framework, including expanded generation of expert fiery cytokines.

When directed to patients or research facility creatures, cytokines have been found to incite regular side effects of misery. Along these lines, a few instances of a low state of mind, low vitality, and absence of inspiration might be because of raised degrees of cytokine proteins.

Vagus Nerve Stimulation (VNS) Dramatically Reduces Arthritic Inflammation

As of late, a global group of specialists from Amsterdam and the United States led a clinical preliminary which exhibits that invigorating the vagus nerve with a little embedded gadget essentially decreased aggravation and improved results for patients with rheumatoid joint pain by repressing cytokine generation.

RA is a constant provocative ailment that influences roughly 1.3 million individuals in the United States and costs several billions of dollars to treat every year, as per the analysts.

The neuroscientists and immunology specialists engaged with this examination utilized best in class innovation to delineate neural hardware that manages irritation. In one circuit—named "the incendiary reflex"— activity possibilities transmitted in the vagus nerve repress the generation of provocative professional cytokines.

The July 2016 investigation, "Vagus Nerve Stimulation Inhibits Cytokine Production and Attenuates Disease Severity in Rheumatoid Arthritis," seems online in the Proceedings of the National Academy of Sciences (PNAS) and will be distributed in an up and coming print issue.

This is the principal human investigation intended to decrease side effects of rheumatoid joint pain by invigorating the vagus nerve with a little embedded gadget which set off a chain response that diminished cytokine levels and irritation. In spite of the fact that this investigation concentrated on rheumatoid joint pain, the preliminary's outcomes may have suggestions for patients experiencing other provocative infections, including Parkinson's, Crohn's, and Alzheimer's.

In an announcement, Paul-Peter Tak, the global head specialist and lead creator of the paper from the Division of Clinical Immunology and Rheumatology of the Academic Medical Center at the University of Amsterdam, stated,

"This is the primary investigation to assess in the case of animating the provocative reflex straightforwardly with an embedded electronic gadget can treat RA in people. We have recently demonstrated that focusing on the incendiary reflex may decrease aggravation in creature models and in vitro models of RA . . . which may be pertinent for other insusceptible interceded incendiary infections too."

These discoveries propose another way to deal with battling infections that are at present treated with moderately costly medications that have a large group of symptoms. VNS gives medicinal services suppliers a possibly increasingly viable approach to improve the lives of individuals experiencing ceaseless provocative ailments.

How improving your vagal tone can prevent physical inflammation

Aggravation is basic to battle contaminations, and yet, it is a significant clinical test in present-day prescription, adding to various sicknesses, including sepsis. In spite of the fact that sepsis is regularly begun by a disease, serious sepsis stays a significant clinical test in present-day prescription, killing more than 250,000 Americans consistently, notwithstanding the viability of the new anti-toxins. Notwithstanding the disease, extreme sepsis is additionally portrayed by the exuberant creation of incendiary cytokines that reason inconvenient fundamental aggravation. New anti-infection agents are progressively viable in controlling diseases, yet they don't control pernicious irritation. Among the incendiary cytokines, Tumor Necrosis Factor (TNF) is a basic factor managing the natural resistant reactions to disease or injury. In any case, inordinate TNF generation turns out to be riskier than the first contamination and causes foundational aggravation, cardiovascular stun, and deadly numerous organ disappointment in sepsis. The hindrance of TNF generation counteracts septic stun, organ harm and improves endurance in test endotoxemia, bacteremia, and sepsis. TNF isn't just created during diseases, and it likewise assumes a basic job in numerous aseptic provocative issues, for example, rheumatoid joint inflammation. Notwithstanding TNF, sepsis is likewise portrayed by the creation of other provocative factors, for example, interleukin IL6 and interferon INF-γ that add to fundamental irritation and various organ disappointment. In this way, late endeavors center around examining the components managing the generation of numerous incendiary elements and their potential clinical interpretation for the treatment of irresistible and provocative issues.

Epidemiological examinations show that physical exercise is among the most significant elements controlling the resistant framework and improving personal satisfaction. Exercise diminishes the danger of numerous conditions, including cardiovascular ailments, hypertension, atherosclerosis, metabolic disorder, diabetes, joint pain, pneumonic issue, dementia, and different kinds of diseases. Long haul normal exercise avoids metabolic and safe issues, yet it's anything but an achievable choice for patients with horribleness or constrained versatility. In this way, late examinations center around the components actuated by exercise to control irritation and their potential clinical interpretation for treating the irresistible and fiery issue. Most investigations on practice center around high-power or long haul standard exercise that causes metabolic pressure or physiological adjustment). Serious anaerobic exercise instigates metabolic pressure, including hypoglycemia, while long haul preparing incites physiological adjustment improving resting pulse, respiratory sinus arrhythmia, cardiovascular vagal tone, and safe guideline. Long haul ordinary preparing seems to manage the safe framework by inciting metabolic and epigenetic versatile instruments. Customary exercise decreases instinctive fat mass, and in this way, forestalls scatter related to heftiness. Accordingly, long haul preparing can likewise counteract aggravation by diminishing the creation of adipokines, provocative variables delivered by adipocytes and fat tissue. In like manner, customary preparing likewise initiates versatile epigenetic alterations in resistant and non-insusceptible tissue, decreasing the generation of provocative factors in monocytes, macrophages. To be sure, competitors have noteworthy lower resting levels of fiery biomarkers including TNF and IL6.

Here are hardly any stunts I've learned throughout the years alongside a couple of key arrangements from the MELT Method that legitimately help with reestablishing perfect vagal tone:

Scrub down in the first part of the day. I know, I know cold showers toward the beginning of the day sound like torment to a few, however, this is an old Chinese cure that helps invigorate the vagus nerve. Generally, what's known as a "hot and cold dive" where you sit in heated water than in a virus dive for 5 minutes each or in any event, placing your face in ice water for 20 seconds and rehashing it 5-10 times additionally are exceptionally viable in vagal incitement.

Sing, giggle, embrace. This appears to be a bit "kumbaya" to a few, yet as the truism goes, chuckling is the best prescription, and an embrace makes you feel much improved. In addition, giggling builds beta-endorphins, nitric oxide, and advantages the vascular framework in general, so spend time with individuals who top you off with affection, chuckling, and generosity. Each of the three likewise discharges oxytocin and serotonin, which are pressure alleviating hormones imperative to our prosperity. What's more, who needn't bother with an embrace? Based on ebb and flow information on neuroanatomy and research with heart vagal tone, I would propose the vagal circuit is connected to feeling guidelines. The vagal circuit of feeling guideline consolidates parallel cerebrum work with the guideline of the fringe autonomic sensory system in the declaration of feeling. Basically, individuals can get asocial if the vagus nerve is disabled or in chaos.

Deal with your gut. The enteric sensory system—or what is portrayed now and then as the gut's sensory system—interface with the mind through the vagus nerve. There is expanding proof indicating an impact of the gut microbiota on the mind. Creatures enhanced with L. rhamnosus experienced different positive changes in GABA receptors that were intervened by the vagus nerve. Eat right, squeeze, and take probiotics to keep your gut vegetation steady and sound. Additionally, irregular fasting or lessening calories has been appeared to build the high-recurrence pulse inconstancy, which is a marker of vagal tone.

Modify pulse inconstancy. This is so easy to do. In The MELT Method, there is something I call the Rebalance Sequence. It is a 10-minute succession that straightforwardly expands HR inconstancy and enables an individual to control a key component of the autonomic sensory system through an astute diaphragmatic method I call the 3-D Breath Breakdown. By backing off and concentrating on the course of diaphragmatic movement, you change the manner in which the brainstem flag the stomach to contract as it does approximately 25,000 times each day when you inhale and don't consider it. At that point, including another procedure called the 3-D Breath, helps the profound center reflex to go enthusiastically, likewise animating vagal tone.

Lessen jaw pressure. The jaw is identified with both the trigeminal and vagus nerve, and the misalignment of the jaw can cause a low vagal tone. On the off chance that you have had supports, loads of mouth work, or have insecure hips and poor foot quality and honesty, you are in danger for low vagal tone. Who knew? All things considered, in my long periods of creating Hands-Off Bodywork, I've made basic at-home methods for my customers with the low vagal tone, and jaw gives that work quick. One is the thing that we call the fast in and out facelift. I shared it on the Rachael Ray Show as an approach to lift the skin around the eyes and mouth, yet I initially built up this strategy for my customers with jaw torment. You can do it anyplace, and it works quick. By animating the tissue where the vagus nerve fans out behind the ears, you can diminish the pressure the tissue regularly has at the base of the skull. This is regularly a guilty party to vagal issues missed in treatment. Now and again, the nerve is, in reality, fine, yet the tissue encompassing it makes lopsided characteristics in its association from mind-gut. By discharging the tissues here with either this method or the neck discharge grouping, you can rapidly help the equalization and association the vagus nerve needs to work productively.

Decompress your neck. The MELT Neck Release Sequence can without much of a stretch decline worry in your body, diminish pointless joint pressure, and straightforwardly impacts vagal tone rapidly. Discharging neck pressure with this straightforward succession additionally lessens strong strain in the chest area where the nerve stretches out at the neck space.

Dissolve your hands and feet. Presently, this is too straightforward. Treat your hands and feet to a MELT treatment as regularly as consistently to reenact the liquid stream all through the whole connective tissue framework just as the billions of tangible nerve endings found in your grasp and feet. The focuses we pack on the hands and feet all identify with locales of the middle, most explicitly our organs. So this is an aberrant method to enable the autonomic sensory system to reestablish entire body balance in as meager as 10 minutes every day.

Chapter Seven: Vagus nerve stimulation routine you can add to your daily habit

The most effective method to begin reconnecting the vagus nerve: it's straightforward, simple, and fun!

Pick a couple of things to begin adding to your day by day schedule – start straightforward, and check whether invigorating the vagus nerve can turn out to be a piece of your human services propensities!

1. Sing. Noisily! Not a calm murmur, yet an all-out, top of your lungs great ole chime in. I prescribe the shower for this one.

The muscles in the back of your throat initiate the vagus nerve as they move, so sing as uproarious as could be expected under the circumstances. Try not to stress over the neighbors.

Oxytocin, the quieting hormone discharged during childbirth, is likewise discharged when we sing.

2. Rinse. You can utilize standard separated water for this. I'm an admirer of proficiency, so I do this in the shower as well. I have a water channel on my shower. So I can believe that the water I'm washing is perfect, and the chlorine has been expelled (which my hair and skin and lungs express gratitude toward me for, as well). When that conditioner is in my hair and doing its enchantment, I wash like an all-out Muppet. Not a careful, exquisite swish – the rinse of a little and-accommodating beast.

You need to swish hard enough that your eyes begin to water

The additional advantage of this is it makes me giggle, and chuckling is an astounding prescription! For this situation, chuckling animates the vagus nerve, as well. Giggling builds beta-endorphins and nitric oxide and advantages of the vascular framework.

It's a success win. What's more, my hair looks Amazing.

3. Work in someday by day petition and contemplation, particularly reciting. It might feel senseless or odd from the start; however it's useful for your wellbeing and health, as what vibrates the throat animates the vagus nerve. It honestly doesn't make a difference what you serenade, simply get to it.

4. Open yourself to cold water or air. The vagus nerve is animated when the body is presented to cold. The thoughtful battle/flight framework is downregulated (works less), and the parasympathetic rest/digest framework is upregulated or requested to work more to quiet you.

5. Do yoga. Both the parasympathetic sensory system and the vagus nerve are animated by yoga practice, especially the Sun Salutation. (

An investigation that looked at a gathering of individuals who strolled day by day to those doing yoga every day found a critical decrease in tension and saw the worry in the yoga gathering, just as increments in the disposition improving, hostile to uneasiness cerebrum synthetic GABA.

6. Ruminate. Reflection and profound breathing animate the vagus nerve.

7. Inhale Deeply and Slowly. There are neurons in both the heart and the neck that contain baroreceptors, or cells that screen your circulatory strain, and send a flag to and fro with your mind.

At the point when we take profound, slow tummy breaths, we actuate the vagus nerve to bring down battle or flight, and initiate our rest and overview parasympathetic sensory system, subsequently bringing down heart rate, circulatory strain, and sentiment of uneasiness.

By and large, we take 10 to 14 breaths for each moment – yet to animate the vagus nerve, attempt to take just six breaths for every moment. Take in profoundly, enabling your stomach to extend, at that point, inhale out gradually.

8. Serotonin and 5HTP. The synapse compound Serotonin enacts the vagus nerve through a wide

range of receptors in the cerebrum, gut, and all through the body. When there is aggravation in the gut, the measure of serotonin made in the cerebrum is diminished by means of the quinoline pathway.

The ideal approach to help ideal mind-body science is started by understanding what is happening in your gut. We can utilize progressed utilitarian prescription stool and breath tests to assess the gut microbiome to perceive what might be causing irritation for you. This is something I accomplish for every one of my patients, particularly those with stomach related problems, despondency, nervousness, skin concerns, hormone awkward nature or rest issues.

Taking the serotonin forerunner 5HTP can help with fundamental serotonin support. This enhancement can associate with certain meds, so make certain to converse with your authorized medicinal services supplier before beginning 5HTP

9. Include Prebiotic and Probiotic nourishments and enhancements. The expression "gut

microbiome" alludes to a great many microorganisms in our stomach related tract, which assumes a job in supplement assimilation, state of mind, hormone, and synapse equalization to give some examples of crucial capacities. The strength of our microbiome is a gigantic determinant of our general wellbeing.

In particular, the probiotic bacterial strain Lactobacillus rhamnosus was appeared in the creature concentrates on helping ideal degrees of the receptors of the quieting compound GABA, which is interceded by the vagus nerve.

For additional on aged nourishments, look at these plans (sauerkraut, beet kvass) for moderate probiotics you can make at home.

Prebiotics, nourishment for the colon cells, are found in stringy vegetables. Go for at least six servings of an assortment of vegetables every day to advance the soundness of your gut, microbiome, colon and vagus nerve.

10. Exercise. At the point when we move, the stomach related framework is invigorated, and the

peristaltic wave, which moves stool through the colon, is additionally actuated.

This development is controlled to a limited extent by the vagus nerve, which is additionally animated by work out, from strolling to yoga to Crossfit.

Whatever activity or development works for you is the proper thing to begin with. Attempt to get some delicate development day by day

11. Needle therapy. People have been invigorating the vagus nerve with needle therapy for a very long time, and there are a few usually utilized focuses that animate improved vagus work.

12. Eat fish! Studies show that consuming omega three unsaturated fats (like those found in greasy fish like salmon) increments vagal tone and movement and places us into that parasympathetic quieting mode all the more frequently.

13. Get a back rub. Kneading various pieces of the body, particularly the feet or along the carotid sinus (on the ride side of your neck), which you can do without anyone else for nothing, can likewise

animate the vagus nerve. Back rub is regularly used to get infants to put on weight since it animates their vagus nerves, subsequently expanding their gut work.

14. Attempt Intermittent Fasting. Research shows that fasting may increment vagal tone also. Fasting may sound threatening, yet it is effectively practiced by basically having supper around 6-7 pm and afterward not having again until breakfast at 7 or 8 am – that is a 13-14 hour quick in that spot! Or then again, you can pack your eating into an 8-10 hour window, state 9 am-7 pm, for a significantly longer quick.

It is an obvious fact that uneasiness and fits of anxiety have an immediate connection with circulatory strain. Presently whether pulse spikes cause uneasiness or tension causes spikes in circulatory strain are still undetermined, and for the most part, episodic. However, there is unquestionably a connection between the two.

The vagus nerve interfaces with various organs in your body, and when not invigorated, can make a scope of issues from uneasiness stomach issues. Having a low vagal tone, which means the nerve isn't animated, could be the reason behind your uneasiness or fits of anxiety. It probably won't be the immediate reason on the grounds that, once more, the vagus nerve is answerable for sending and accepting sign from the remainder of your body. On the off chance that your uneasiness is brought about by gut issues, at that point, animating your vagus nerve could expand your vagal tone, and thusly, perhaps help your gut issue.

How can one increment vagal tone? Many express that everything from profound breathing to singing expands your vagal tone by sending a sign to your vagus nerve through quite certain neurons whose activity is to identify and bring down circulatory strain and pulse. These are incredible techniques for invigorating the vagus nerve and ought to be utilized related to the best strategy for expanding your parasympathetic sensory system: ice.

Ice

Uncovering your vagus nerve to cold conditions is the quickest and best technique for rapidly closing down the body's battle or-flight reaction that is causing the tension or fit of anxiety. Putting an ice pack on the back of your neck will expand your parasympathetic sensory system and quiets you down very quickly by bringing down your pulse.

You can accomplish considerably increasingly outrageous vagal nerve incitement by hopping into a virus shower or sprinkling your face with super cold water while taking full breaths.

So whenever you feel your furthest points depleting, your chest getting tight, and a tension assault going ahead — go after an ice pack from your cooler, place it on the back of your neck, and take full breaths. You can physically feel your body quieting itself down. Contingent upon the reason for your tension, this strategy over the intellectual, social treatment may end the assaults for good.

Chapter Eight: How to strengthen Vagus Nerve

Four Ways to Strengthen Your Stress Resilience

Yoga Self-Care

What makes a few of us ricochet back despite life's difficulties, and others disintegrate? Why is it that, a few days, we feel ready to take on the world, while on different days, one seemingly insignificant detail can set us off? There are, without a doubt, various responses to these inquiries be that as it may, on a physiological level, analysts realize that our pressure strength levels are associated with a certain something: the vagus nerve.

The vagus nerve, our tenth cranial nerve, adjusts the parasympathetic sensory system, the piece of the sensory system that causes us to quiet down and unwind. Likewise called the "meandering nerve" since it wanders through the body, the vagus nerve directs heart and breath rate and controls our voice tone, organs, and stomach related tract. From multiple points of view, the vagus nerve is the air traffic controller of our physical body—sending and getting messages from the cerebrum about when to process, when to inhale, and what to feel. This makes it a fundamental player in building pressure versatility.

Strangely, the condition of our vagus nerve can be estimated. Researchers built up a measure called pulse fluctuation, which tracks the time between heart pulsates. When there is changeability between heart thumps, this suggests a high vagal tone, which is associated with great pressure flexibility. When there is a little fluctuation between heart thumps, this suggests a low vagal tone, which is related to poor pressure versatility. The primary concern? When there is adaptability in our pulses, as opposed to an inflexible beating, we are stronger. Sounds entirely like yoga, isn't that so? Adaptability implies versatility and improved general wellbeing.

Fortunately, the vagus nerve can be reinforced through the way of life, practice, and aim. Here are a couple of practices that have been appeared to increment vagal tone.

Slow, Deep, Breathing

This training is, without a doubt probably the most ideal approaches to improve the quality of the vagus nerve. Researchers contend this is one motivation behind why yoga is so amazing—due to the accentuation on the breath. It encourages us to unwind by initiating the vagus nerve and supporting our sensory system. Slow stomach breathing can improve vagal tone. Likewise, Ocean-Sounding Breath (Ujjayi pranayama), in which you make a delicate narrowing in the back of your throat, can additionally upgrade the advantages. The vagus nerve contacts the throat, so making a tad of rubbing in the throat as you inhale can help invigorate the vagus and improve vagal tone. Have a go at delaying during work to inhale profoundly for a couple of seconds, and notice how you feel.

Exercise

Moderate to concentrated exercise has been appeared to improve pulse inconstancy, the marker of vagal tone. Studies show that normal exercise in sound grown-ups, just as grown-ups with cardiovascular illness, improved vagal tone. The exercise doesn't need to be long-only 20 minutes can have an effect. While look into this has not yet been done, it would appear to pursue that consolidating yogic breathing with moderate exercise would additionally upgrade the impacts of pressure versatility and vagal tone.

Metta Meditation

Metta reflection, otherwise called cherishing thoughtfulness contemplation, is simply the act of sending kind considerations to yourself as well as other people. Scientist Barbara Fredrickson found that Metta's contemplation improved vagal tone for some who rehearsed it. She contrasted a control bunch with those rehearsing Metta and found that when individuals revealed increments in warm and cherishing sentiments, their vagal tone improved.

Have a go at rehearsing Metta contemplation as you nod off; not exclusively will you improve your vagal tone, you may likewise be emphatically affecting your fantasy life, as per the Buddhist writings.

Brief Recitation

An examination demonstrated that reciting om can improve vagal tone by invigorating the nerves around the throat. On the off chance that om isn't your thing, you can likewise have a go at singing noisily—what the hell, nobody's tuning in the vehicle. Feel the reverberation in your throat and all through your body.

Plainly yoga offers an assortment of apparatuses to increment vagal tone and along these lines, bolster pressure flexibility. The key is to rehearse at least one of these instruments every day, regardless of whether it's only for five minutes. Also, recall, it sets aside an effort to fortify the sensory system, yet persistence and practice can carry us to a progressively adjusted condition of being.

The vagus nerve is really a basket case driving from the gut through the heart and to the cerebrum. It's the longest cranial nerve and has correspondence with each organ.

Its fundamental capacity is to control the parasympathetic sensory system. The parasympathetic sensory system is a piece of the autonomic help framework known as the "rest and overview" framework. It assumes a job in pulse, sexual excitement, absorption, pee, and gastrointestinal action.

The vagus nerve works enthusiastically to control irritation. It alarms the cerebrum to discharge synapses when provocative proteins called cytokines are available. These synapses help the body fix at that point decrease aggravation.

Another capacity of the vagus nerve is to trigger the arrival of acetylcholine, which controls muscles, enlarges veins, and eases back pulse. It's sheltered to state the vagus nerve might be the most significant nerve that most of the individuals are as yet ignorant of.

Researchers have connected vagus nerve brokenness to heftiness, constant aggravation, wretchedness, uneasiness, seizures, unusually low pulse, blacking out, and GI issues.

Actually, the examination on this nerve has been promising to the point that vagus nerve triggers have been embedded in patients and discovered achievement even with untreatable sadness and epilepsy. The gadget is carefully embedded under the skin and sends an electrical sign to the vagus nerve. When invigorated, the vagus nerve begins speaking with the remainder of the body.

Fortunate for us, there's no requirement for medical procedures. Vagal tone can be improved normally through incitement with systems that should be possible at home. Attempting to reinforce your vagal tone will help with state of mind, processing, and general prosperity.

Nineteen efficient ways to Improve Vagal Tone

1. Swishing. This is presumably the least complex and most open route for an individual to chip away at their vagal tone. In the first part of the day, wash some water as hard as possible. You'll realize you've invigorated the vagus nerve when you start to get a tear reaction in your eyes.

2. Breathwork. Profound moderate breaths from the tummy will animate the vagus nerve. Sit or sit down and take in as much as you can. Hold it for a second or two and afterward discharge. Rehash this 5-10 times. You'll feel euphoric and lose a while later.

3. Giggling. Giggling discharges a huge amount of synapse, which improves vagal tone. Giggle hard and regularly.

4. Fish Oils. EPA and EHA lower pulse, which reinforces the vagal tone.

5. Fasting. The vagus nerve is the chief of the parasympathetic sensory system known as the rest

and condensation framework. Offering the assimilation procedure a reprieve through discontinuous fasting or fewer snacks for the duration of the day will likewise improve vagal tone.

6. Yoga. The breathing and development of yoga assist with absorption and has been appeared to build GABA levels. Improving GABA levels will animate the vagal tone.

7. Singing. Singing works the muscles in the back of the throat, which invigorates the vagus nerve. Simply make certain to sing as loud as possible for this impact to occur. An extraordinary spot to do this is in the vehicle.

8. Cold Showers. Cold showers are extreme from the start, yet they can enormously improve vagal tone. As you change in accordance with the cool, the thoughtful sensory system brings down, and the parasympathetic framework gets more grounded, legitimately influencing the vagus nerve.

9. Backrub. A back rub invigorates the lymphatics and improves the vagal tone.

10. Fragrance based treatment. Fundamental oils, for example, lavender and bergamot, have appeared to expand pulse inconstancy, which improves vagal tone.

11. Developing Positive Relationships

Research shows that just by thinking about our friends and family, we can tone and reinforce the vagus nerve, consequently receiving the numerous rewards that the nerve gives.

12. Presentation to the Cold

By drinking cold water or washing up, we reinforce our body's quieting framework (the parasympathetic framework), which occurs through the vagus nerve.

13. singing and Chanting

Singing as loud as possible expands pulse inconstancy and works the muscles in the back of your throat that associate with the vagus nerve.

14. Back rubs

Apart from feeling astounding, a great back rub of the feet and neck actives the vagus nerve and can diminish seizures.

15. Satisfaction and Laughter

Having a decent snicker lifts your mind-set, supports the insusceptible framework, and animates the vagus nerve.

16. Yoga and Tai Chi

Both Yoga and Tai Chi give a large group of medical advantages and are especially useful for those battling with wretchedness and nervousness.

17. Profound Breathing

Profound breathing animates the vagus nerve to bring down circulatory strain and pulse.

18. Exercise

Physical exercise is ground-breaking both for gut stream and psychological well-being benefits, which both happen by means of the vagus nerve.

19. Unwinding

Practically any loosening up action reinforces the vegas nerve's capacity to give recuperating to the body.

Therefore, these are ways that can help strengthen the vagal tone for you.

Printed in the USA
CPSIA information can be obtained
at www.ICGtesting.com
LVHW040345040724
784655LV00014B/133